NANDA-I | NURSING DIAGNOSES:
DEFINITIONS & CLASSIFICATION
2007–2008

D1365064

Editorial Committee

T. Heather Herdman, PhD, RN, *Chair*
Crystal Heath, MSN, RN
Geralyn Meyer, PhD, RN
Leann Scroggins, MN, RN, CCRN-A, APRN BC
Barbara Vassallo, EdD, RN, CS, ANPC

Managing Editor: Margo C. Neal

NANDA-I

NURSING DIAGNOSES:
DEFINITIONS &
CLASSIFICATION
2007–2008

NANDA International
Philadelphia

This edition, *NANDA-I Nursing Diagnosis: Definitions & Classification 2007–2008*, supercedes all previous editions.

For information, contact NANDA International,
100 North 20th Street, Philadelphia PA 19103, USA
Telephone: 215.545.7222 / 800.647.9002
Fax: 215.564.2175
E-mail: info@nanda.org
Web: www.nanda.org

Printed in the United States of America
10 9 8 7 6 5 4 3 2 1

ISBN 978-0-9788924-0-1

Contents

Preface

The *NANDA-I Nursing Diagnoses: Definitions & Classification 2007-2008* edition contains the most revisions and additions of nursing diagnoses to the NANDA-International taxonomy in many years. We are pleased to announce the addition of 15 new diagnoses, as well as 26 revised diagnoses. The new diagnoses reflect an emphasis on health promotion and add two community-focused diagnoses: *Contamination* and *Risk for Contamination*. Four of the accepted revisions to diagnoses were submitted from individuals outside of the United States (Brazil and Canada), which is reflective of the increasing internationalization of nursing diagnosis terminology. The Board of Directors continues to encourage participation from all countries to enable the continuing utilization and applicability of nursing diagnosis terminology globally.

You will notice that in this edition almost every diagnosis has some changes to its defining characteristics and related or risk factors. The concepts have not changed but, to enable ease of coding, they have been separated and/or condensed as we begin to use the same word to define concepts (e.g., "dyspnea" rather than "shortness of breath"). We have begun this work in this edition and anticipate that we will continue to refine the diagnoses in the next edition. We ask you to bear with us as we complete this important work; it is a fitting reminder that our language is growing and changing as our knowledge advances.

Other changes in this edition include the addition of information on the use and applicability of nursing diagnoses within nursing education, nursing informatics, nursing research, and nursing administration. This information is offered as a brief introduction on the importance of nursing diagnoses to each of these critical areas within the nursing profession, particularly due to the increased interest being expressed by individuals in those areas who are beginning to see the need to look beyond the more obvious clinical applicability of the nursing diagnoses.

Because of the increased awareness of the need for standardized nursing language to name what nurses do, to allow its presence to be captured and its effects measured through information systems, I want to encourage those of you who are not currently members of NANDA-International to take the time now to join our organization. And don't stop there—bring along a peer, a student, a manager, a nurse informaticist! All of our patients will benefit from the wisdom of the voices of nurses from a variety of practice areas and backgrounds. The Invitation to Join NANDA-International is found on page 335.

It is important to note that many of the revised and new diagnoses came about as a direct result of increased activity by the members of the Diagnosis Review Committee (DRC). Almost one half (12) of the revised diagnoses and two of the new diagnoses were developed by members of this committee in response to the call from the Board of Directors for a proactive role for the committee, in addition to its established role in the review of incoming submissions. It is anticipated that this level of activity will continue as the DRC becomes the Diagnosis Development Committee within the new governance structure of NANDA-International. However, it is also important to emphasize that these diagnoses are held to the same standard as any submitter's work. Diagnoses must be clearly supported through research evidence; we provide this evidence via the Level of Evidence (LOE) number assigned to each new and revised diagnosis to indicate the exact extent of underlying scientific evidence that exists for each diagnosis.

We are, once again, providing the diagnoses in alphabetical order *by diagnostic concept*. We have heard some concerns from members of the global community that this is not always helpful for non-English speaking users, and for that we must certainly apologize. However, to date we have not identified another method of organizing the diagnoses that has been agreed upon universally. We certainly encourage you to contact NANDA-International with recommendations that would make this book more user-friendly in the future.

This book would not be possible without the continued commitment of an extraordinary individual who agreed to continue her involvement with it as its managing editor, Margo Neal. I want to thank her for her willingness to continue with this work and for making the publication of this book possible. I also want to extend my sincere gratitude to the members of the editorial committee, whose hard work also enabled the publication of this edition. Finally, I want to thank all of you who have developed and submitted diagnoses and/or revisions to NANDA-International this cycle, and all of those of you who came before. Without your dedication to standardized nursing language, there would be nothing at all to publish. We have jumped from 172 diagnoses to 188 with this edition, but this is simply not enough to describe the richness of nursing practice.

I would like to issue a challenge to each and every one of you to commit to developing and submitting one revision or one new diagnosis to NANDA-International's Diagnosis Development Committee over the next two year cycle. Can you imagine how much more representative the taxonomy of nursing practice would be if each of us accepted that challenge? I urge you to do just that—find that one crucial diagnosis you always regret is missing and develop it! Or, take the diagnosis that is long overdue for an update, make it better, and send it in! Contact Leann Scroggins, Chair of the Diagnosis Development Committee, to be assigned a mentor to guide you through this process (she can be reached through NANDA-I's Web site). Or, log on to www.nlinks.org and use the tools provided there to develop your concept analysis. The submission guidelines are presented in this book for you to see (page 320), and are also available on our Web site: www.nanda.org. What are you waiting for? There is plenty to do, and you are just the person to do it—we look forward to your submission to NANDA-International's Diagnosis Development Committee.

T. Heather Herdman, PhD, RN
President, NANDA International

New Nursing Diagnoses, 2007-2008

Contamination
Laura Polk, DNSc, RN, & Pauline Green, PhD, RN
Moral Distress
Lisa Burkhart, PhD, MPH, RN, &
Beverly Kopala, PhD, RN
Overflow Urinary Incontinence
Geralyn Meyer, PhD, RN
Readiness for Enhanced Comfort
Readiness for Enhanced Decision Making
Readiness for Enhanced Hope
Readiness for Enhanced Immunization Status
Readiness for Enhanced Power
Readiness for Enhanced Self-Care
Margaret Lunney, PhD, RN,
Roberta Cavendish, PhD, RN, CPN,
Barbara Kraynyak Luise, EdD, RN, &
Kathryn Richardson, MA, RN
Risk for Acute Confusion
Peggy Stimpert, MSN, RN
Risk for Contamination
Laura Polk, DNSc, RN, & Pauline Green, PhD, RN
Risk for Compromised Human Dignity
Susan Rosenberg, MSN, RN, CNRN, CHI
Risk for Impaired Liver Function
Kathryn White, BSN, MT, RN
Risk for Unstable Blood Glucose
Janice Denehy, PhD, RN
Stress Overload
Margaret Lunney, PhD, RN

Revised Nursing Diagnoses, 2007-2008

Acute Confusion
    Diagnosis Development Committee
Complicated Grieving (previously titled "*Dysfunctional Grieving*")
    T. Heather Herdman, PhD, RN
Death Anxiety
    Amor Aradilla, MS, RN, Lidia Fernández, MS, RN,
    Pilar Fernández, MS, RN, & Joaquín Tomás, PhD, RN
Decisional Conflict
    Lisa Burkhart, PhD, RN, & Beverly Kopala, PhD, RN
Delayed Surgical Recovery
    Susan Kleinbeck, PhD, RN, CNOR
Grieving (previously titled "*Anticipatory Grieving*")
    T. Heather Herdman, PhD, RN
Latex Allergy Response
    Susan Kleinbeck, PhD, RN, CNOR
Impaired Bed Mobility
Impaired Transfer Ability
    Meridean Maas, PhD, RN, FAAN
Impaired Urinary Elimination
    Lynda Carpenito-Moyet, MSN, RN, CRNP
Impaired Walking
Impaired Wheelchair Mobility
    Meridean Maas, PhD, RN, FAAN
Ineffective Denial
    Lina Rahal, MEd, RN, & Vivianne Saba, MSN, RN
Ineffective Infant Feeding Pattern
    Lynda Carpenito-Moyet, MSN, RN, CRNP
Ineffective Sexuality Pattern
    Alexandra Souza Melo, PhD, RN,
    Emilia Campos de Carvalho, PhD, RN, &
    Nilza Tereza Rotter Pelá, PhD, RN
Insomnia (previously titled "disturbed sleep pattern")
    Aleita White, MSN, RN

Risk for Complicated Grieving (previously titled "risk for dysfunctional grieving")
   T. Heather Herdman, PhD, RN
Risk for Latex Allergy Response
   Susan Kleinbeck, PhD, RN, CNOR
Risk for Loneliness
   Lynda Carpenito-Moyet, MSN, RN, CRNP
Risk for Perioperative Positioning Injury
   Susan Kleinbeck, PhD, RN, CNOR
Risk for Poisoning
   Laura Polk, DNSc, RN, & Pauline Green, PhD, RN
Risk-Prone Health Behavior (previously titled "Impaired Adjustment")
   Micky Gonzales, MSN, NP-C
Sexual Dysfunction
   Alexandra Souza Melo, PhD, RN,
   Emilia Campos de Carvalho, PhD, RN, &
   Nilza Tereza Rotter Pelá, PhD, RN
Stress Urinary Incontinence
   Geralyn Meyer, PhD, RN
Unilateral Neglect
   Ibtihal Almakhzoomy, MSN, RN, Lina Rahal, MEd, RN,
   Danielle Schmouth, MEd, RN &
   Genevieve Lefrancois, MSN, RN
Urge Urinary Incontinence
   Geralyn Meyer, PhD, RN

Introduction

This book is divided into three parts. Part 1 includes the traditional contents of the previous *NANDA Nursing Diagnoses: Definitions & Classification* books—that is, the diagnoses. The diagnoses are listed in *alphabetical order by the diagnostic concept,* not by the first word or descriptor of the diagnosis. Thus, if you are looking for *impaired wheelchair mobility,* you will find it under "mobility," not under "wheelchair" or "impaired."

Taxonomy II splits the diagnoses into axes (see page 255 for a full explanation). Part 2 describes the structure of Taxonomy II and how it was developed. Figure 2.1 depicts *Taxonomy II Domains and Classes;* Table 2.1 shows *Taxonomy II: Domains, Classes, and Diagnoses;* and Table 2.2 shows *NNN Taxonomy of Nursing Practice: Placement of Nursing Diagnoses.*

Part 3 includes information on how nursing diagnoses are used in the areas of administration, education, informatics, and research. As well, this part contains diagnosis submission guidelines, a process to appeal a decision of the Diagnosis Development Committee, and a glossary; a list of members of the NANDA International Board of Directors, Taxonomy and Diagnosis Development Committees; an invitation to join NANDA-I; and the index.

How to Use This Book

As noted above, the nursing diagnoses are listed alphabetically by *diagnostic concept.* For example, *activity intolerance* is listed under "A" because activity is the diagnostic concept. Similarly, *interrupted family process* is listed under "F" because family process is the diagnostic concept.

We hope the organization of *NANDA-I Nursing Diagnoses: Definitions & Classification 2007–2008* will make it efficient and effective to use. We welcome your feedback. If you have suggestions, please send them to us through the NANDA-I Web site (http://www.nanda.org) or by calling the office at 800. 647.9002.

NANDA Guidelines for Copyright Permission

The materials presented in this book are copyrighted and all copyright laws apply. Situations requiring approvals and/or copyright fees are listed below:

1. An author or publishing house requests use of the entire nursing diagnosis taxonomy in a textbook or other nursing manual to be sold.
2. An author or publishing house requests use of only the list of nursing diagnoses with no definitions or defining characteristics.
3. An author or company requests use of the nursing diagnosis taxonomy in an audiovisual material.
4. A software developer or computer-based patient record vendor requests use of the nursing diagnosis taxonomy in a program.
5. A nursing school, researcher, professional organization, or healthcare organization requests use of the nursing diagnosis taxonomy in a program.

Send all permission requests to:
NANDA International
100 N. 20th Street/4th Floor
Philadelphia, PA 19103, USA
Telephone: 800.647.9002/215.545.8105
fax: 215.564.2175
e-mail: info@nanda.org
Web: www.nanda.org

Part 1

NANDA-I NURSING DIAGNOSES 2007–2008

ACTIVITY INTOLERANCE
(1982)

Definition *Insufficient physiological or psychological energy to endure or complete required or desired daily activities*

Defining Characteristics
- Abnormal blood pressure response to activity
- Abnormal heart rate response to activity
- Electrocardiographic changes reflecting arrhythmias
- Electrocardiographic changes reflecting ischemia
- Exertional discomfort
- Exertional dyspnea
- Verbal report of fatigue
- Verbal report of weakness

Related Factors
Bed rest
Generalized weakness
Imbalance between
  oxygen supply/demand
Immobility
Sedentary lifestyle

RISK FOR ACTIVITY INTOLERANCE
(1982)

Definition   *At risk for experiencing insufficient physiological or psychological energy to endure or complete required or desired daily activities*

Risk Factors

Deconditioned status

History of previous intolerance

Inexperience with the activity

Presence of circulatory problems

Presence of respiratory problems

INEFFECTIVE AIRWAY CLEARANCE
(1980, 1996, 1998)

Definition *Inability to clear secretions or obstructions from the respiratory tract to maintain a clear airway*

Defining Characteristics

- Absent cough
- Adventitious breath sounds
- Changes in respiratory rate
- Changes in respiratory rhythm
- Cyanosis
- Difficulty vocalizing
- Diminished breath sounds
- Dyspnea
- Excessive sputum
- Ineffective cough
- Orthopnea
- Restlessness
- Wide-eyed

Related Factors

Environmental

Second-hand smoke
Smoke inhalation
Smoking

Obstructed airway

Airway spasm
Excessive mucus
Exudate in the alveoli
Foreign body in airway
Presence of artificial airway
Retained secretions
Secretions in the bronchi

Physiological

Allergic airways
Asthma
Chronic obstructive pulmonary disease
Hyperplasia of the bronchial walls
Infection
Neuromuscular dysfunction

LATEX ALLERGY RESPONSE
(1998, 2006, LOE 2.1)

Definition *A hypersensitive reaction to natural latex rubber products*

Defining Characteristics

Life-Threatening Reactions Occurring < 1 Hour After Exposure to Latex Protein

- Bronchospasm
- Cardiac arrest
- Contact urticaria progressing to generalized symptoms
- Dyspnea
- Edema of the lips
- Edema of the throat
- Edema of the tongue
- Edema of the uvula
- Hypotension
- Respiratory arrest
- Syncope
- Tightness in chest
- Wheezing

Orofacial Characteristics

- Edema of eyelids
- Edema of sclera
- Erythema of the eyes
- Facial erythema
- Facial itching
- Itching of the eyes
- Oral itching
- Nasal congestion
- Nasal erythema
- Nasal itching
- Rhinorrhea
- Tearing of the eyes

Gastrointestinal Characteristics

- Abdominal pain
- Nausea

Generalized Characteristics

- Flushing
- Generalized discomfort
- Generalized edema
- Increasing complaint of total body warmth
- Restlessness

Type 1V Reactions Occurring > 1 Hour After Exposure to Latex Protein

- Discomfort reaction to additives such as thiurams & carbamates
- Eczema
- Irritation
- Redness

Related Factors

Hypersensitivity to
natural latex rubber
protein

References

American Society of Anesthesiologists. (2005). *Natural rubber latex allergy:Considerations for anesthesiologists* (a practice guideline). Park Ridge, IL: Author.

AORN. (2004). AORN latex guideline. In *AORN standards, recommended practices and guidelines* (pp. 103–118). Denver, CO: Author.

Sussman, G.L. (2000) Latex allergy: An overview. *Canadian Journal of Allergy and Clinical Immunology, 5,* 317–321.

RISK FOR LATEX ALLERGY RESPONSE
(1998, 2006, LOE 2.1)

Definition *Risk of hypersensitivity to natural latex rubber products*

Risk Factors

Allergies to avocados
Allergies to bananas
Allergies to chestnuts
Allergies to kiwi
Allergies to poinsettia plants
Allergies to tropical fruits
History of allergies
History of asthma
History of reactions to latex
Multiple surgical procedures, especially from infancy
Professions with daily exposure to latex

References

American Society of Anesthesiologists. (2005). *Natural rubber latex allergy:Considerations for anesthesiologists* (a practice guideline). Park Ridge, IL: Author.

AORN. (2004). AORN latex guideline. In *AORN standards, recommended practices and guidelines* (pp. 103–118). Denver, CO: Author.

Sussman, G.L. (2000) Latex allergy: An overview. *Canadian Journal of Allergy and Clinical Immunology, 5,* 317–321.

ANXIETY
(1973, 1982, 1998)

Definition   *Vague uneasy feeling of discomfort or dread accompanied by an autonomic response (the source often non-specific or unknown to the individual); a feeling of apprehension caused by anticipation of danger. It is an alerting signal that warns of impending danger and enables the individual to take measures to deal with threat.*

Defining Characteristics

Behavioral
- Diminished productivity
- Expressed concerns due to change in life events
- Extraneous movement
- Fidgeting
- Glancing about
- Insomnia
- Poor eye contact
- Restlessness
- Scanning
- Vigilance

Affective
- Apprehensive
- Anguish
- Distressed
- Fearful
- Feelings of inadequacy
- Focus on self
- Increased wariness
- Irritability
- Jittery
- Overexcited
- Painful increased helplessness
- Persistent increased helplessness
- Rattled
- Regretful
- Scared
- Uncertainty
- Worried

Physiological
- Facial tension
- Hand tremors
- Increased perspiration
- Increased tension
- Shakiness
- Trembling
- Voice quivering

Sympathetic
- Anorexia
- Cardiovascular excitation
- Diarrhea
- Dry mouth
- Facial flushing
- Heart pounding
- Increased blood pressure
- Increased pulse
- Increased reflexes

continued

Anxiety, *continued*

- Increased respiration
- Pupil dilation
- Respiratory difficulties
- Superficial vasoconstriction
- Twitching
- Weakness

Parasympathetic

- Abdominal pain
- Decreased blood pressure
- Decreased pulse
- Diarrhea
- Faintness
- Fatigue
- Nausea
- Sleep disturbance
- Tingling in extremities
- Urinary frequency
- Urinary hesitancy
- Urinary urgency

Cognitive

- Awareness of physiologic symptoms
- Blocking of thought
- Confusion
- Decreased perceptual field
- Difficulty concentrating
- Diminished ability to learn
- Diminished ability to problem solve
- Fear of unspecified consequences
- Forgetfulness
- Impaired attention
- Preoccupation
- Rumination
- Tendency to blame others

Related Factors

Change in
– Economic status
– Environment
– Health status
– Interaction patterns
– Role function
– Role status
Exposure to toxins
Familial association
Heredity
Interpersonal contagion
Interpersonal transmission
Maturational crises
Situational crises
Stress

Substance abuse
Threat of death
Threat to
– Economic status
– Environment
– Health status
– Interaction patterns
– Role function
– Role status
Threat to self-concept
Unconscious conflict about essential goals of life
Unconscious conflict about essential values
Unmet needs

DEATH ANXIETY
(1998, 2006, LOE 2.1)

Definition *Vague uneasy feeling of discomfort or dread generated by perceptions of a real or imagined threat to one's existence*

Defining Characteristics

- Reports concerns of over-working the caregiver
- Reports deep sadness
- Reports fear of developing terminal illness
- Reports fear of loss of mental abilities when dying
- Reports fear of pain related to dying
- Reports fear of premature death
- Reports fear of the process of dying
- Reports fear of prolonged dying
- Reports fear of suffering related to dying
- Reports feeling powerless over dying
- Reports negative thoughts related to death and dying
- Reports worry about the impact of one's own death on significant others

Related Factors

Anticipating adverse consequences of general anesthesia
Anticipating impact of death on others
Anticipating pain
Anticipating suffering
Confronting reality of terminal disease
Discussions on topic of death
Experiencing dying process

Near death experience
Nonacceptance of own mortality
Observations related to death
Perceived proximity of death
Uncertainty about an encounter with a higher power

continued

Death Anxiety, *continued*

Uncertainty about the
existence of a higher
power

Uncertainty about life
after death
Uncertainty of prognosis

References

Abdel-Khalek, A., & Tomàs-Sàbado, J. (2005). Anxiety and death anxiety in Egyptian and Spanish nursing students. *Death Studies, 29,* 157-169.

Bay, E., & Algase, D. (1999). Fear and anxiety: A simultaneous concept analysis. *Nursing Diagnosis, 10,* 103-11.

Kastenbaum, R. (1992). *The psychology of death.* New York: The Guliford Press

RISK FOR ASPIRATION
(1988)

Definition   *At risk for entry of gastrointestinal secretions, oropharyngeal secretions, solids, or fluids into tracheobronchial passages*

Risk Factors

Decreased gastrointestinal motility
Delayed gastric emptying
Depressed cough
Depressed gag reflex
Facial surgery
Facial trauma
Gastrointestinal tubes
Incompetent lower esophageal sphincter
Increased gastric residual
Increased intragastric pressure
Impaired swallowing
Medication administration
Neck trauma
Neck surgery
Oral surgery
Oral trauma
Presence of endotracheal tube
Presence of tracheostomy tube
Reduced level of consciousness
Situations hindering elevation of upper body
Tube feedings
Wired jaws

RISK FOR IMPAIRED PARENT/CHILD ATTACHMENT
(1994)

Definition *Disruption of the interactive process between parent/significant other and child/infant that fosters the development of a protective and nurturing reciprocal relationship*

Risk Factors

Anxiety associated with the parent role

Ill infant/child who is unable to effectively initiate parental contact due to altered behavioral organization

Inability of parents to meet personal needs

Lack of privacy

Parental conflict due to altered behavioral organization

Physical barriers

Premature infant who is unable to effectively initiate parental contact due to altered behavioral organization

Separation

Substance abuse

Autonomic Dysreflexia
(1988)

Definition *Life-threatening, uninhibited sympathetic response of the nervous system to a noxious stimulus after a spinal cord injury at T7 or above*

Defining Characteristics

- Blurred vision
- Bradycardia
- Chest pain
- Chilling
- Conjunctival congestion
- Diaphoresis (above the injury)
- Headache (a diffuse pain in different portions of the head and not confined to any nerve distribution area)
- Horner's syndrome
- Metallic taste in mouth
- Nasal congestion
- Pallor (below the injury)
- Paresthesia
- Paroxysmal hypertension
- Pilomotor reflex
- Red splotches on skin (above the injury)
- Tachycardia

Related Factors

Bladder distention
Bowel distention
Deficient caregiver knowledge
Deficient patient knowledge
Skin irritation

RISK FOR Autonomic Dysreflexia
(1998, 2000)

Definition *At risk for life-threatening, uninhibited response of the sympathetic nervous system, post spinal shock, in an individual with spinal cord injury or lesion at T6 or above (has been demonstrated in patients with injuries at T7 and T8)*

Risk Factors

An injury at T6 or above or a lesion at T6 or above AND at least one of the following noxious stimuli:

Cardiac/Pulmonary Problems
- Deep vein thrombosis
- Pulmonary emboli

Gastrointestinal Stimuli
- Bowel distention
- Constipation
- Difficult passage of feces
- Digital stimulation
- Enemas
- Esophageal reflux
- Fecal impaction
- Gallstones
- Gastric ulcers
- GI system pathology
- Hemorrhoids
- Suppositories

Musculoskeletal-Integumentary Stimuli
- Cutaneous stimulation (e.g., pressure ulcer, ingrown toenail, dressings, burns, rash)
- Fractures
- Heterotrophic bone

- Pressure over bony prominences
- Pressure over genitalia
- Range-of-motion exercises
- Spasm
- Sunburns
- Wounds

Neurological Stimuli
- Irritating stimuli below level of injury
- Painful stimuli below level of injury

Regulatory Stimuli
- Extreme environmental temperatures
- Temperature fluctuations

Reproductive Stimuli
- Ejaculation
- Labor and delivery
- Menstruation
- Ovarian cyst
- Pregnancy
- Sexual intercourse

Situational Stimuli

- Constrictive clothing (e.g., straps, stockings, shoes)
- Drug reactions (e.g., decongestants, sympathomimetics, vasoconstrictors)
- Narcotic withdrawal
- Positioning
- Surgical procedure

Urological Stimuli

- Bladder distention
- Bladder spasm
- Calculi
- Catheterization
- Cystitis
- Detrusor sphincter dysynergia
- Epididymitis
- Instrumentation
- Surgery
- Urethritis
- Urinary tract infection

B

RISK-PRONE HEALTH BEHAVIOR*
(1986, 1998, 2006, LOE 2.1)

Definition *Inability to modify lifestyle/behaviors in a manner consistent with a change in health status*

Defining Characteristics

- Demonstrates nonacceptance of health status change
- Failure to achieve optimal sense of control
- Failure to take action that prevents health problems
- Minimizes health status change

Related Factors

Inadequate comprehension

Inadequate social support

Low self-efficacy

Low socioeconomic status

Multiple stressors

Negative attitude toward health care

References

Kiefe C.L., Heudebert G., Box J.B., Farmer R.M., Micahel M., & Clancy C.M. (1999). Compliance with post-hospitalization follow-up visits: Rationing by inconvenience? *Ethnicity & Disease, 19,* 387–395.

Koenigsberg, M., Barlett, D., & Carmer, J. (2004). Facilitating treatment adherence with lifestyle changes in diabetes. *American Family Physician, 69,* 309–316, 319–320, 323–324..

Shemesh, E. (2004). Non-adherence to medications following pediatric liver transplantation. *Pediatric Transplantation, 8,* 600–605.

Previously titled "Impaired Adjustment"

DISTURBED **B**ODY IMAGE
(1973, 1998)

Definition   *Confusion in mental picture of one's physical self*

Defining Characteristics

- Behaviors of acknowl-edgment of one's body
- Behaviors of avoidance of one's body
- Behaviors of monitoring one's body
- Nonverbal response to actual change in body (e.g., appearance, struc-ture, or function)
- Nonverbal response to perceived change in body (e.g., appearance, struc-ture, or function)
- Verbalization of feelings that reflect an altered view of one's body (e.g., appearance, structure, function)
- Verbalization of percep-tions that reflect an altered view of one's body in appearance

Objective

- Actual change in function
- Actual change in structure
- Behaviors of acknowl-edging one's body
- Behaviors of monitoring one's body
- Change in ability to esti-mate spatial relationship of body to environment
- Change in social involve-ment
- Extension of body boundary to incorporate environmental objects
- Intentional hiding of body part
- Intentional overexposure of body part
- Missing body part
- Not looking at body part
- Not touching body part
- Trauma to nonfunction-ing part
- Unintentional hiding of body part
- Unintentional overexpos-ing of body part

Subjective

- Depersonalization of loss by impersonal pronouns
- Depersonalization of part by impersonal pronouns
- Emphasis on remaining strengths
- Fear of reaction by others

continued

B

Disturbed Body Image, *continued*

- Fear of rejection by others
- Focus on past appearance
- Focus on past function
- Focus on past strength
- Heightened achievement
- Negative feelings about body (e.g., feelings of helplessness, hopelessness, or powerlessness)
- Personalization of loss by name
- Personalization of part by name
- Preoccupation with change
- Preoccupation with loss
- Refusal to verify actual change
- Verbalization of change in lifestyle

Related Factors

Biophysical
Cognitive
Cultural
Developmental changes
Illness
Illness treatment

Injury
Perceptual
Psychosocial
Spiritual
Surgery
Trauma

RISK FOR IMBALANCED BODY TEMPERATURE
(1986, 2000)

Definition   *At risk for failure to maintain body temperature within normal range*

Risk Factors

Altered metabolic rate
Dehydration
Exposure to cold/cool
  environments
Exposure to warm/hot
  environments
Extremes of age
Extremes of weight
Illness affecting tempera-
  ture regulation
Inactivity

Inappropriate clothing
  for environmental
  temperature
Medications causing
  vasoconstriction
Medications causing
  vasodilation
Sedation
Trauma affecting temper-
  ature regulation
Vigorous activity

B

Bowel incontinence
(1975, 1998)

Definition *Change in normal bowel habits characterized by involuntary passage of stool*

Defining Characteristics

- Constant dribbling of soft stool
- Fecal odor
- Fecal staining of bedding
- Fecal staining of clothing
- Inability to delay defecation
- Inability to recognize urge to defecate
- Inattention to urge to defecate
- Recognizes rectal fullness but reports inability to expel formed stool
- Red perianal skin
- Self-report of inability to recognize rectal fullness
- Urgency

Related Factors

Abnormally high abdominal pressure
Abnormally high intestinal pressure
Chronic diarrhea
Colorectal lesions
Dietary habits
Environmental factors (e.g., inaccessible bathroom)
General decline in muscle tone
Immobility
Impaired cognition
Impaired reservoir capacity
Incomplete emptying of bowel
Laxative abuse
Loss of rectal sphincter control
Lower motor nerve damage
Medications
Rectal sphincter abnormality
Impaction
Stress
Toileting self-care deficit
Upper motor nerve damage

EFFECTIVE BREASTFEEDING
(1990)

Definition   *Mother-infant dyad/family exhibits adequate proficiency and satisfaction with breastfeeding process*

Defining Characteristics

- Adequate infant elimination patterns for age
- Appropriate infant weight pattern for age
- Eagerness of infant to nurse
- Effective mother/infant communication patterns
- Infant content after feeding
- Maternal verbalization of satisfaction with the breastfeeding process
- Mother able to position infant at breast to promote a successful latching-on response
- Regular and sustained suckling at the breast
- Regular and sustained swallowing at the breast
- Signs of oxytocin release
- Symptoms of oxytocin release

Related Factors

Basic breastfeeding knowledge
Infant gestational age >34 weeks
Maternal confidence
Normal breast structure
Normal infant oral structure
Support source

B

INEFFECTIVE BREASTFEEDING
(1988)

Definition *Dissatisfaction or difficulty a mother, infant, or child experiences with the breastfeeding process*

Defining Characteristics

- Inadequate milk supply
- Infant arching at the breast
- Infant crying at the breast
- Infant inability to latch on to maternal breast correctly
- Infant exhibiting crying within the first hour after breastfeeding
- Infant exhibiting fussiness within the first hour after breastfeeding
- Insufficient emptying of each breast per feeding
- Insufficient opportunity for suckling at the breast
- No observable signs of oxytocin release
- Nonsustained suckling at the breast
- Observable signs of inadequate infant intake
- Perceived inadequate milk supply
- Persistence of sore nipples beyond first week of breastfeeding
- Resisting latching on
- Unresponsive to other comfort measures
- Unsatisfactory breastfeeding process

Related Factors

Infant anomaly
Infant receiving supplemental feedings with artificial nipple
Interruption in breastfeeding
Knowledge deficit
Maternal ambivalence
Maternal anxiety

Maternal breast anomaly
Nonsupportive family
Nonsupportive partner
Poor infant sucking reflex
Prematurity
Previous breast surgery
Previous history of breastfeeding failure

INTERRUPTED **B**REASTFEEDING
(1992)

Definition *Break in the continuity of the breastfeeding process as a result of inability or inadvisability to put baby to breast for feeding*

Defining Characteristics

- Infant receives no nour-ishment at the breast for some or all feedings
- Lack of knowledge regarding expression of breast milk
- Lack of knowledge regarding storage of breast milk
- Maternal desire to even-tually provide breast milk for infant/child's nutritional needs
- Maternal desire to main-tain breastfeeding for infant/child's nutritional needs
- Maternal desire to pro-vide breast milk for infant/child's nutritional needs
- Separation of mother and infant

Related Factors

Contraindications to breastfeeding
Infant illness
Maternal employment
Maternal illness
Need to abruptly wean infant
Prematurity

B

INEFFECTIVE BREATHING PATTERN
(1980, 1996, 1998)

Definition *Inspiration and/or expiration that does not provide adequate ventilation*

Defining Characteristics

- Alterations in depth of breathing
- Altered chest excursion
- Assumption of 3-point position
- Bradypnea
- Decreased expiratory pressure
- Decreased inspiratory pressure
- Decreased minute ventilation
- Decreased vital capacity
- Dyspnea
- Increased anterior-posterior diameter
- Nasal flaring
- Orthopnea
- Prolonged expiration phase
- Pursed-lip breathing
- Tachypnea
- Timing ratio
- Use of accessory muscles to breathe

Related Factors

Anxiety
Body position
Bony deformity
Chest wall deformity
Cognitive impairment
Fatigue
Hyperventilation
Hypoventilation syndrome
Musculoskeletal impairment

Neurological immaturity
Neuromuscular dysfunction
Obesity
Pain
Perception impairment
Respiratory muscle fatigue
Spinal cord injury

DECREASED CARDIAC OUTPUT
(1975, 1996, 2000)

Definition *Inadequate blood pumped by the heart to meet metabolic demands of the body*

Defining Characteristics

Altered Heart Rate/ Rhythm

- Arrhythmias
- Bradycardia
- EKG changes
- Palpitations
- Tachycardia

Altered Preload

- Edema
- Decreased central venous pressure (CVP)
- Decreased pulmonary artery wedge pressure (PAWP)
- Fatigue
- Increased central venous pressure (CVP)
- Increased pulmonary artery wedge pressure (PAWP)
- Jugular vein distention
- Murmurs
- Weight gain

Altered Afterload

- Clammy skin
- Dyspnea
- Decreased peripheral pulses
- Decreased pulmonary vascular resistance (PVR)
- Decreased systemic vascular resistance (SVR)
- Increased pulmonary vascular resistance (PVR)
- Increased systemic vascular resistance (SVR)
- Oliguria
- Prolonged capillary refill
- Skin color changes
- Variations in blood pressure readings

Altered Contractility

- Crackles
- Cough
- Decreased ejection fraction
- Decreased left ventricular stroke work index (LVSWI)
- Decreased stroke volume index (SVI)

continued

Decreased Cardiac Output, *continued*

C

- Decreased cardiac index
- Decreased cardiac output
- Orthopnea
- Paroxysmal nocturnal dyspnea
- S3 sounds
- S4 sounds

Behavioral/Emotional
- Anxiety
- Restlessness

Related Factors

Altered heart rate
Altered rhythm

Altered Stroke Volume

Altered afterload
Altered contractility
Altered preload

CAREGIVER ROLE STRAIN
(1992, 1998, 2000)

Definition *Difficulty in performing family caregiver role*

Defining Characteristics

Caregiving Activities

- Apprehension about care receiver's care if caregiver unable to provide care
- Apprehension about the future regarding care receiver's health
- Apprehension about the future regarding caregiver's ability to provide care
- Apprehension about possible institutionalization of care receiver
- Difficulty completing required tasks
- Difficulty performing required tasks
- Dysfunctional change in caregiving activities
- Preoccupation with care routine

Caregiver Health Status

Physical

- Cardiovascular disease
- Diabetes
- Fatigue
- GI upset
- Headaches
- Hypertension
- Rash
- Weight change

Emotional

- Anger
- Disturbed sleep
- Feeling depressed
- Frustration
- Impaired individual coping
- Impatience
- Increased emotional lability
- Increased nervousness
- Lack of time to meet personal needs
- Somatization
- Stress

Socioeconomic

- Changes in leisure activities
- Low work productivity
- Refuses career advancement
- Withdraws from social life

continued

C

Caregiver Role Strain, *continued*

Caregiver-Care Receiver Relationship

- Difficulty watching care receiver go through the illness
- Grief regarding changed relationship with care receiver

- Uncertainty regarding changed relationship with care receiver

Family Processes

- Concerns about family members
- Family conflict

Related Factors

Care Receiver Health Status

Addiction
Codependency
Cognitive problems
Dependency
llness chronicity
Illness severity
Increasing care needs
Instability of care receiver's health
Problem behaviors
Psychological problems
Unpredictability of illness course

Caregiver Health Status

Addiction
Codependency
Cognitive problems
Inability to fulfill one's own expectations
Inability to fulfill other's expectations
Marginal coping patterns
Physical problems

Psychological problems
Unrealistic expectations of self

Caregiver-Care Receiver Relationship

History of poor relationship
Mental status of elder inhibiting conversation
Presence of abuse
Presence of violence
Unrealistic expectations of caregiver by care receiver

Caregiving Activities

24-hour care responsibilities
Amount of activities
Complexity of activities
Discharge of family members to home with significant care needs
Ongoing changes in activities

C

Unpredictability of care situation

Years of caregiving

Family Processes

History of family dysfunction

History of marginal family coping

Resources

Caregiver is not developmentally ready for caregiver role

Deficient knowledge about community resources

Difficulty accessing community resourses

Emotional strength

Formal assistance

Formal support

Inadequate community resources (e.g., respite services, recreational resources)

Inadequate equipment for providing care

Inadequate physical environment for providing care (e.g., housing, temperature, safety)

Inadequate transportation

Inexperience with caregiving

Informal assistance

Informal support

Insufficient finances

Insufficient time

Lack of caregiver privacy

Lack of support

Physical energy

Socioeconomic

Alienation from others

Competing role commitments

Insufficient recreation

Isolation from others

C RISK FOR CAREGIVER ROLE STRAIN
(1992)

Definition *Caregiver is vulnerable for felt difficulty in performing the family caregiver role*

Risk Factors

Addiction

Amount of caregiving tasks

Care receiver exhibits bizarre behavior

Care receiver exhibits deviant behavior

Caregiver's competing role commitments

Caregiver health impairment

Caregiver is female

Caregiver is spouse

Caregiver isolation

Caregiver not developmentally ready for caregiver role

Codependency

Cognitive problems in care receiver

Complexity of caregiving tasks

Congenital defect

Developmental delay of the care receiver

Developmental delay of the caregiver

Discharge of family member with significant home care needs

Duration of caregiving required

Family dysfunction prior to the caregiving situation

Family isolation

Illness severity of the care receiver

Inadequate physical environment for providing care (e.g., housing, transportation, community services, equipment)

Inexperience with caregiving

Instability in the care receiver's health

Lack of recreation for caregiver

Lack of respite for caregiver

Marginal caregiver's coping patterns

Marginal family adaptation

Past history of poor relationship between caregiver and care receiver

Premature birth

C

Presence of abuse

Presence of situational stressors that normally affect families (e.g., significant loss, disaster or crisis, economic vulnerability, major life events)

Presence of violence

Psychological problems in care receiver

Retardation of the care receiver

Retardation of the caregiver

Unpredictable illness course

C

READINESS FOR ENHANCED COMFORT
(2006, LOE 2.1)

Definition *A pattern of ease, relief, and transcendence in physical, psychospiritual, environmental, and/or social dimensions that can be strengthened*

Defining Characteristics
- Expresses desire to enhance comfort
- Expresses desire to enhance feeling of contentment
- Expresses desire to enhance relaxation
- Expresses desire to enhance resolution of complaints

References

Duggleby, W., & Berry, P. (2005). Transitions in shifting goals of care for palliative patients and their families. *Clinical Journal of Oncology Nursing, 9,* 425–428.

Kolcaba, K. (1994). A theory of holistic comfort for nursing. *Journal of Advanced Nursing, 19,* 1178–1184.

Malinowski, A., & Stamler, L.L. (2002). Comfort: Exploration of the concept in nursing. *Journal of Advanced Nursing, 39,* 599–606.

IMPAIRED VERBAL COMMUNICATION
(1983, 1996, 1998)

Definition   *Decreased, delayed, or absent ability to receive, process, transmit, and/or use a system of symbols*

Defining Characteristics

- Absence of eye contact
- Cannot speak
- Difficulty in comprehending usual communication pattern
- Difficulty expressing thoughts verbally (e.g., aphasia, dysphasia, apraxia, dyslexia)
- Difficulty forming sentences
- Difficulty forming words (e.g., aphonia, dyslalia, dysarthria)
- Difficulty in maintaining usual communication pattern
- Difficulty in selective attending
- Difficulty in use of body expressions
- Difficulty in use of facial expressions
- Disorientation to person
- Disorientation to space
- Disorientation to time
- Does not speak
- Dyspnea
- Inability to speak language of caregiver
- Inability to use body expressions
- Inability to use facial expressions
- Inappropriate verbalization
- Partial visual deficit
- Slurring
- Speaks with difficulty
- Stuttering
- Total visual deficit
- Verbalizes with difficulty
- Willful refusal to speak

Related Factors

Absence of significant others
Altered perceptions
Alteration in self-concept
Alteration in self-esteem
Alteration of central nervous system

continued

C

Impaired Verbal Communication, *continued*

Anatomical defect (e.g., cleft palate, alteration of the neuromuscular visual system, auditory system, phonatory apparatus)

Brain tumor

Cultural differences

Decrease in circulation to brain

Differences related to developmental age

Emotional conditions

Environmental barriers

Lack of information

Physical barrier (e.g., tracheostomy, intubation)

Physiological conditions

Psychological barriers (e.g., psychosis, lack of stimuli)

Side effects of medication

Stress

Weakening of the musculoskeletal system

READINESS FOR ENHANCED COMMUNICATION
(2002, LOE 2.1)

Definition *A pattern of exchanging information and ideas with others that is sufficient for meeting one's needs and life's goals, and can be strengthened*

Defining Characteristics

- Able to speak a language
- Able to write a language
- Expresses feelings
- Expresses satisfaction with ability to share ideas with others
- Expresses satisfaction with ability to share information with others
- Expresses thoughts
- Expresses willingness to enhance communication
- Forms phrases
- Forms sentences
- Forms words
- Interprets nonverbal cues appropriately
- Uses nonverbal cues appropriately

C

DECISIONAL CONFLICT
(1988,2006, LoE 2.1)

Definition *Uncertainty about course of action to be taken when choice among competing actions involves risk, loss, or challenge to values and beliefs*

Defining Characteristics

- Delayed decision making
- Physical signs of distress or tension (e.g., increased heart rate, increased muscle tension, restlessness)
- Questioning moral principles while attempting a decision
- Questioning moral rules while attempting a decision
- Questioning moral values while attempting a decision
- Questioning personal beliefs while attempting a decision
- Questioning personal values while attempting a decision
- Self-focusing
- Vacillation among alternative choices
- Verbalizes feeling of distress while attempting a decision
- Verbalizes uncertainty about choices
- Verbalizes undesired consequences of alternative actions being considered

Related Factors

Divergent sources of information
Interference with decision making
Lack of experience with decision making
Lack of relevant information

Moral obligations require performing action
Moral obligations require not performing action
Moral principles support mutually inconsistent courses of action

C

Moral rules support mutually inconsistent courses of action
Moral values support mutually inconsistent courses of action
Multiple sources of information

Perceived threat to value system
Support system deficit
Unclear personal beliefs
Unclear personal values

References

Beauchamp, T., & Childress, J. (2001). *Principles of biomedical ethics* (5th ed.). New York: Oxford University Press.

Kopala, B., & Burkhart, L. (2005). Ethical dilemma and moral distress: Proposed new NANDA diagnoses. *International Journal of Nursing Terminologies and Classifications, 16,* 3–13.

Webster, G., & Baylis, F. (2000). Moral residue. In S. Rubin & L. Zoloth (Eds.), *Margin of error. The ethics of mistakes in the practice of medicine* (pp. 217–230). Hagerstown, MD: University Publishing.

C

PARENTAL ROLE CONFLICT
(1988)

Definition *Parent experience of role confusion and conflict in response to crisis*

Defining Characteristics

- Anxiety
- Demonstrated disruption in caretaking routines
- Expresses concern about perceived loss of control over decisions relating to their child
- Fear
- Parent(s) express(es) concern(s) about changes in parental role
- Parent(s) express(es) concern(s) about family (e.g., functioning, communication, health)
- Parent(s) express(es) concern(s) of inadequacy to provide for child's needs (e.g., physical, emotional)
- Parent(s) express(es) feeling(s) of inadequacy to provide for child's needs (e.g., physical, emotional)
- Reluctant to participate in usual caretaking activities even with encouragement and support
- Verbalizes feelings of frustration
- Verbalizes feelings of guilt

Related Factors

Change in marital status
Home care of a child with special needs
Interruptions of family life due to home care regimen (e.g., treatments, caregivers, lack of respite)
Intimidation with invasive modalities (e.g., intubation)
Intimidation with restrictive modalities (e.g., isolation)
Separation from child due to chronic illness
Specialized care center

ACUTE CONFUSION
(1994, 2006, LOE 2.1)

Definition *Abrupt onset of reversible disturbances of consciousness, attention, cognition, and perception that develop over a short period of time*

Defining Characteristics
- Fluctuation in cognition
- Fluctuation in level of consciousness
- Fluctuation in psychomotor activity
- Hallucinations
- Increased agitation
- Increased restlessness
- Lack of motivation to follow through with goal-directed behavior
- Lack of motivation to follow through with purposeful behavior
- Lack of motivation to initiate goal-directed behavior
- Lack of motivation to initiate purposeful behavior
- Misperceptions

Related Factors
Alcohol abuse
Delirium
Dementia
Drug abuse
Fluctuation in sleep-wake cycle
Over 60 years of age

References

Schor, J., Levkoff, S., Lipsitz, L., Reilly, C., Cleary, P., Rowe, J., et al. (1992). Risk factors for delirium in hospitalized elderly. *JAMA, 267*, 827–831.

Inouye, S., & Charpentier, P. (1996). Precipitating factors for delirium in hospitalized elderly persons: Predictive model and interrelationship with baseline vulnerability. *JAMA, 275*, 852–857.

Inouye, S., Viscoli, C., Horwitz, R., Hurst, L., & Tinetti, M. (1993). A predictive model for delirium in hospitalized elderly medical patients based on admission characteristics. *Archives of Internal Medicine, 119*, 474–481.

C

CHRONIC CONFUSION
(1994)

Definition *Irreversible, long-standing, and/or progressive deterioration of intellect and personality characterized by decreased ability to interpret environmental stimuli; decreased capacity for intellectual thought processes; and manifested by disturbances of memory, orientation, and behavior*

Defining Characteristics

- Altered interpretation
- Altered personality
- Altered response to stimuli
- Clinical evidence of organic impairment
- Impaired long-term memory
- Impaired short-term memory
- Impaired socialization
- Long-standing cognitive impairment
- No change in level of consciousness
- Progressive cognitive impairment

Related Factors

Alzheimer's disease
Cerebral vascular attack
Head injury
Korsakoff's psychosis
Multi-infarct dementia

RISK FOR ACUTE Confusion

(2006, LOE 2.2)

Definition   *At risk for reversible disturbances of consciousness, attention, cognition, and perception that develop over a short period of time*

Risk Factors

Alcohol use

Decreased mobility

Decreased restraints

Dementia

Fluctuation in sleep-wake
  cycle

History of stroke

Impaired cognition

Infection

Male gender

Medication/Drugs
  – Anesthesia
  – Anticholinergics
  – Diphenhydramine
  – Multiple medications
  – Opoids
  – Psychoactive drugs

Metabolic abnormalities
  – Azotemia
  – Decreased hemoglobin
  – Dehydration
  – Electrolyte imbalances
  – Increased
    BUN/Creatinine
  – Malnutrition

Over 60 years of age

Pain

Sensory deprivation

Substance abuse

Urinary retention

References

Schor, J., Levkoff, S., Lipsitz, L., Reilly, C., Cleary, P., Rowe, J., et al. (1992). Risk factors for delirium in hospitalized elderly. *JAMA, 267,* 827–831.

Inouye, S., & Charpentier, P. (1996). Precipitating factors for delirium in hospitalized elderly persons: Predictive model and interrelationship with baseline vulnerability. *JAMA, 275,* 852–857.

Inouye, S., Viscoli, C., Horwitz, R., Hurst, L., & Tinetti, M. (1993). A predictive model for delirium in hospitalized elderly medical patients based on admission characteristics. *Archives of Internal Medicine, 119,* 474–481.

C **CONSTIPATION**
(1975, 1998)

Definition *Decrease in normal frequency of defecation accompanied by difficult or incomplete passage of stool and/or passage of excessively hard, dry stool*

Defining Characteristics

- Abdominal pain
- Abdominal tenderness with palpable muscle resistance
- Abdominal tenderness without palpable muscle resistance
- Anorexia
- Atypical presentations in older adults (e.g., change in mental status, urinary incontinence, unexplained falls, elevated body temperature)
- Borborygmi
- Bright red blood with stool
- Change in bowel pattern
- Decreased frequency
- Decreased volume of stool
- Distended abdomen
- Feeling of rectal fullness
- Feeling of rectal pressure
- Generalized fatigue
- Hard, formed stool
- Headache
- Hyperactive bowel sounds
- Hypoactive bowel sounds
- Increased abdominal pressure
- Indigestion
- Nausea
- Oozing liquid stool
- Palpable abdominal mass
- Palpable rectal mass
- Presence of soft, paste-like stool in rectum
- Percussed abdominal dullness
- Pain with defecation
- Severe flatus
- Straining with defecation
- Unable to pass stool
- Vomiting

Related Factors

Functional

Abdominal muscle weakness

Habitual denial

Habitual ignoring of urge to defecate

Inadequate toileting (e.g., timeliness, positioning for defecation, privacy)

Irregular defecation habits

Insufficient physical activity

Recent environmental changes

Psychological

Depression

Emotional stress

Mental confusion

Pharmacological

Aluminum-containing antacids

Anticholinergics

Anticonvulsants

Antidepressants

Antilipemic agents

Bismuth salts

Calcium carbonate

Calcium channel blockers

Diuretics

Iron salts

Laxative overdose

Nonsteroidal antiinflammatory agents

Opiates

Phenothiazines

Sedatives

Sympathomimetics

Mechanical

Electrolyte imbalance

Hemorrhoids

Hirschsprung's disease

Neurological impairment

Obesity

Postsurgical obstruction

Pregnancy

Prostate enlargement

Rectal abscess

Rectal anal fissures

Rectal anal stricture

Rectal prolapse

Rectal ulcer

Rectocele

Tumors

Physiological

Change in eating patterns

Change in usual foods

Decreased motility of gastrointestinal tract

Dehydration

Inadequate dentition

Inadequate oral hygiene

Insufficient fiber intake

Insufficient fluid intake

Poor eating habits

C

PERCEIVED CONSTIPATION
(1988)

Definition *Self-diagnosis of constipation and abuse of laxatives, enemas, and suppositories to ensure a daily bowel movement*

Defining Characteristics

- Expectation of a daily bowel movement
- Expectation of passage of stool at same time every day
- Overuse of laxatives
- Overuse of enemas
- Overuse of suppositories

Related Factors

Cultural health beliefs
Family health beliefs
Faulty appraisal
Impaired thought processes

RISK FOR CONSTIPATION
(1998)

C

Definition *At risk for a decrease in normal frequency of defecation accompanied by difficult or incomplete passage of stool and/or passage of excessively hard, dry stool*

Risk Factors

Functional

Habitual denial/ignoring of urge to defecate
Recent environmental changes
Inadequate toileting (e.g., timeliness, positioning for defecation, privacy)
Irregular defecation habits
Insufficient physical activity
Abdominal muscle weakness

Psychological

Depression
Emotional stress
Mental confusion

Physiological

Change in usual eating patterns
Change in usual foods
Decreased motility of gastrointestinal tract
Dehydration
Inadequate dentition
Inadequate oral hygiene
Insufficient fiber intake
Insufficient fluid intake
Poor eating habits

Pharmacological

Aluminum-containing antacids
Anticholinergics
Anticonvulsants
Antidepressants
Antilipemic agents
Bismuth salts
Calcium carbonate
Calcium channel blockers
Diuretics
Iron salts
Laxative overuse
Nonsteroidal anti-inflammatory agents
Opiates
Phenothiazines
Sedatives
Sympathomimetics

Mechanical

Electrolyte imbalance
Hemorrhoids
Hirschsprung's disease
Neurological impairment
Obesity
Postsurgical obstruction
Pregnancy

continued

C

Risk for Constipation, *continued*

Prostate enlargement
Rectal abscess
Rectal anal fissures
Rectal anal stricture
Rectal prolapse
Rectal ulcer
Rectocele
Tumors

CONTAMINATION

C

(2006, LOE 2.1)

Definition *Exposure to environmental contaminants in doses sufficient to cause adverse health effects*

Defining Characteristics

(Defining characteristics are dependent on the causative agent. Agents cause a variety of individual organ responses as well as systemic responses.)

Pesticides

- Dermatological effects of pesticide exposure
- Gastrointestinal effects of pesticide exposure
- Neurological effects of pesticide exposure
- Pulmonary effects of pesticide exposure
- Renal effects of pesticide exposure

(Major categories of pesticides: Insecticides, herbicides, fungicides, antimicrobials, rodenticides
Major pesticides: organophosphates, carbamates, organochlorines, pyrethrium, arsenic, glycophosphates, bipyridyls, chlorophenoxy)

Chemicals

- Dermatological effects of chemical exposure
- Gastrointestinal effects of chemical exposure
- Immunologic effects of chemical exposure
- Neurological effects of chemical exposure
- Pulmonary effects of chemical exposure
- Renal effects of chemical exposure

(Major chemical agents: petroleum-based agents, anticholinesterases
Type I agents act on proximal tracheobronchial portion of the respiratory tract, Type II agents act on aveoli, Type III agents produce systemic effects)

Biologics

- Dermatological effects of exposure to biologics
- Gastrointestinal effects of exposure to biologics
- Pulmonary effects of exposure to biologics
- Neurological effects of exposure to biologics

continued

C

Contamination, *continued*

• Renal effects of exposure to biologics (toxins from living organisms (bacteria, viruses, fungi))

Pollution

• Neurological effects of pollution exposure
• Pulmonary effects of pollution exposure

(Major locations: Air, water, soil

Major agents: asbestos, radon, tobacco, heavy metal, lead, noise, exhaust)

Waste

• Dermatological effects of waste exposure
• Gastrointestinal effects of waste exposure
• Hepatic effects of waste exposure
• Pulmonary effects of waste exposure

(Categories of waste: trash, raw sewage, industrial waste)

Radiation

• Immunologic effects of radiation exposure
• Genetic effects of radiation exposure
• Neurological effects of radiation exposure
• Oncologic effects of radiation exposure

(Categories: Internal — exposure through ingestion of radioactive material (e.g., food / water contamination)

External — exposure through direct contact with radioactive material)

Related Factors

External

Chemical contamination of food
Chemical contamination of water
Exposure to bioterrorism
Exposure to disaster (natural or man-made)

Exposure to radiation (occupation in radiography, employment in nuclear industries and electrical generating plants, living near nuclear industries and electrical generating plants)

C

Flaking, peeling paint in presence of young children

Flaking, peeling plaster in presence of young children

Flooring surface (carpeted surfaces hold contaminant residue more than hard floor surfaces)

Geographic area (living in area where high level of contaminants exist)

Household hygiene practices

Inadequate municipal services (trash removal, sewage treatment facilities)

Inappropriate use of protective clothing

Lack of breakdown of contaminants once indoors (breakdown is inhibited without sun and rain exposure)

Lack of protective clothing

Living in poverty (increases potential for multiple exposure, lack of access to health care, and poor diet)

Paint, lacquer, etc. in poorly ventilated areas

Paint, lacquer, etc. without effective protection

Personal hygiene practices

Playing in outdoor areas where environmental contaminants are used

Presence of atmospheric pollutants

Use of environmental contaminants in the home (e.g., pesticides, chemicals, environmental tobacco smoke)

Unprotected contact with heavy metals or chemicals (e.g., arsenic, chromium, lead)

Internal

Age (children less than 5 years, older adults)

Concomitant exposures

Developmental characteristics of children

Female gender

Gestational age during exposure

Nutritional factors (e.g., obesity, vitamin and mineral deficiencies)

Pre-existing disease states

Pregnancy

Previous exposures

Smoking

continued

C

Contamination, *continued*

References

Berkowitz, G.S., Obel, J., Deych, E., Lapinski, R., Godbold, J., & Liu, Z. (2003). Exposure to indoor pesticides during pregnancy in a multiethnic, urban cohort. *Environmental Health Perspectives, 111,* 79–84.

Center for Disease Control and Prevention. (2005). Third national report on human exposure to environmental chemicals: Executive summary (NCEH Pub # 05-0725). Atlanta, GA: Author.

McCauley, L.A., Michaels, S., Rothlein, J., Muniz, J., Lasarev, M., & Ebbert, C. (2003). Pesticide exposure and self-reported home hygiene. *AAOHN Journal, 51,* 113–119.

RISK FOR CONTAMINATION
(2006, LOE 2.1)

C

Definition *Accentuated risk of exposure to environmental contaminants in doses sufficient to cause adverse health effects*

Risk Factors

External

Chemical contamination of food

Chemical contamination of water

Exposure to bioterrorism

Exposure to disaster (natural or man-made)

Exposure to radiation (occupation in radiography, employment in nuclear industries and electrical generating plants, living near nuclear industries and electrical generating plants)

Flaking, peeling paint in presence of young children

Flaking, peeling plaster in presence of young children

Flooring surface (carpeted surfaces hold contaminant residue more than hard floor surfaces)

Geographic area (living in area where high level of contaminants exist)

Household hygiene practices

Inadequate municipal services (e.g., trash removal, sewage treatment facilities)

Inappropriate use of protective clothing

Lack of breakdown of contaminants once indoors (breakdown is inhibited without sun and rain exposure)

Lack of protective clothing

Living in poverty (increases potential for multiple exposure, lack of access to health care, and poor diet)

Paint, lacquer, etc. in poorly ventilated areas

Paint, lacquer, etc. without effective protection

Personal hygiene practices

Playing in outdoor areas where environmental contaminants are used

continued

C

Risk for Contamination, *continued*

Presence of atmospheric pollutants

Use of environmental contaminants in the home (e.g., pesticides, chemicals, environmental tobacco smoke

Unprotected contact with heavy metals or chemicals (e.g., arsenic, chromium, lead)

Internal

Age (children less than 5 years, older adults)

Concomitant exposures

Developmental characteristics of children

Female gender

Gestational age during exposure

Nutritional factors (e.g., obesity, vitamin and mineral deficiencies)

Pre-existing disease states

Pregnancy

Previous exposures

Smoking

References

Centers for Disease Control and Prevention. (2005). *Third national report on human exposure to environmental chemicals: Executive summary* (NCEH Pub # 05-0725). Atlanta: Author.

Chalupka, S.M. (2001). Essentials of environmental health. Enhancing your occupational health nursing practice (Part II). *AAOHN Journal, 49,* 194–213.

McCauley, L.A., Michaels, S., Rothlein, J., Muniz, J., Lasarev, M., & Ebbert, C. (2003). Pesticide exposure and self-reported home hygiene. *AAOHN Journal, 51,* 113–119.

COMPROMISED FAMILY CoPING
(1980, 1996)

C

Definition   *Usually supportive primary person (family member or close friend) provides insufficient, ineffective, or compromised support, comfort, assistance, or encouragement that may be needed by the client to manage or master adaptive tasks related to his/her health challenge*

Defining Characteristics

Objective

- Significant person attempts assistive behaviors with unsatisfactory results
- Significant person attempts supportive behaviors with unsatisfactory results
- Significant person displays protective behavior disproportionate to client's abilities
- Significant person displays protective behavior disproportionate to client's need for autonomy
- Significant person enters into limited personal communication with client
- Significant person withdraws from client

Subjective

- Client expresses a complaint about significant other's response to health problem
- Client expresses a concern about significant other's response to health problem
- Significant person expresses an inadequate knowledge base, which interferes with effective supportive behaviors
- Significant person expresses an inadequate understanding, which interferes with supportive behaviors
- Significant person describes preoccupation with personal reaction (e.g., fear, anticipatory grief, guilt, anxiety) to client's need

continued

C

Compromised Family Coping, *continued*

Related Factors

Coexisting situations affecting the significant person

Developmental crises the significant person may be facing

Exhaustion of supportive capacity of significant people

Inadequate information by a primary person

Inadequate understanding of information by a primary person

Incorrect information by a primary person

Incorrect understanding of information by a primary person

Lack of reciprocal support

Little support provided by client, in turn, for primary person

Prolonged disease that exhausts supportive capacity of significant people

Situational crises the significant person may be facing

Temporary family disorganization

Temporary family role changes

Temporary preoccupation by a significant person

DEFENSIVE COPING
(1988)

C

Definition *Repeated projection of falsely positive self-evaluation based on a self-protective pattern that defends against underlying perceived threats to positive self-regard*

Defining Characteristics

- Denial of obvious problems
- Denial of obvious weaknesses
- Difficulty establishing relationships
- Difficulty maintaining relationships
- Difficulty in perception of reality
- Difficulty in perception of reality testing
- Grandiosity
- Hostile laughter
- Hypersensitivity to criticism
- Hypersensitivity to slight
- Lack of follow-through in therapy
- Lack of follow-through in treatment
- Lack of participation in therapy
- Lack of participation in treatment
- Projection of blame
- Projection of responsibility
- Rationalization of failures
- Ridicule of others
- Superior attitude toward others

Related Factors

To be developed

Note. This diagnosis will retire from the NANDA-I Taxonomy in the 2009–2010 edition unless additional work is done to bring it to a LOE of 2.1 or higher.

C

DISABLED FAMILY COPING
(1980, 1996)

Definition *Behavior of significant person (family member or other primary person) that disables his/her capacities and the client's capacities to effectively address tasks essential to either person's adaption to the health challenge*

Defining Characteristics

- Abandonment
- Aggression
- Agitation
- Carrying on usual routines without regard for client's needs
- Client's development of dependence
- Depression
- Desertion
- Disregarding client's needs
- Distortion of reality regarding client's health problem
- Family behaviors that are detrimental to well-being
- Hostility
- Impaired individualization
- Impaired restructuring of a meaningful life for self
- Intolerance
- Neglectful care of client in regard to basic human needs
- Neglectful care of client in regard to illness treatment
- Neglectful relationships with other family members
- Prolonged overconcern for client
- Psychosomaticism
- Rejection
- Taking on illness signs of client

Related Factors

Arbitrary handling of family's resistance to treatment

Dissonant coping styles for dealing with adaptive tasks by the significant person and client

Dissonant coping styles among significant people

Highly ambivalent family relationships

Significant person with chronically unexpressed feelings (e.g., guilt, anxiety, hostility, despair)

INEFFECTIVE COPING
(1978, 1998)

C

Definition *Inability to form a valid appraisal of the stressors, inadequate choices of practiced responses, and/or inability to use available resources*

Defining Characteristics

- Abuse of chemical agents
- Change in usual communication patterns
- Decreased use of social support
- Destructive behavior toward others
- Destructive behavior toward self
- Fatigue
- High illness rate
- Inability to meet basic needs
- Inability to meet role expectations
- Inadequate problem solving
- Lack of goal-directed behavior/resolution of problem, including inability to attend to and difficulty organizing information
- Poor concentration
- Risk taking
- Sleep disturbance
- Use of forms of coping that impede adaptive behavior
- Verbalization of inability to ask for help
- Verbalization of inability to cope

Related Factors

Disturbance in pattern of appraisal of threat

Disturbance in pattern of tension release

Gender differences in coping strategies

High degree of threat

Inability to conserve adaptive energies

Inadequate level of confidence in ability to cope

Inadequate level of perception of control

Inadequate opportunity to prepare for stressor

Inadequate resources available

continued

C

Ineffective Coping, *continued*

Inadequate social sup-
   port created by charac-
   teristics of relationships
Maturational crisis
Situational crisis
Uncertainty

INEFFECTIVE COMMUNITY COPING
(1994, 1998)

Definition   *Pattern of community activities for adaptation and problem solving that is unsatisfactory for meeting the demands or needs of the community*

Defining Characteristics

- Community does not meet its own expectations
- Deficits in community participation
- Excessive community conflicts
- Expressed community powerlessness
- Expressed vulnerability
- High illness rates
- Increased social problems (e.g., homicides, vandalism, arson, terrorism, robbery, infanticide, abuse, divorce, unemployment, poverty, militancy, mental illness)
- Stressors perceived as excessive

Related Factors

Deficits in community social support services
Deficits in community social support resources
Natural disasters
Man-made disasters
Inadequate resources for problem solving
Ineffective community systems (e.g., lack of emergency medical system, transportation system, or disaster planning systems)
Nonexistent community systems

C | READINESS FOR ENHANCED COPING
(2002, LOE 2.1)

Definition *A pattern of cognitive and behavioral efforts to manage demands that is sufficient for well-being and can be strengthened.*

Defining Characteristics
- Acknowledges power
- Aware of possible environmental changes
- Defines stressors as manageable
- Seeks knowledge of new strategies
- Seeks social support
- Uses a broad range of emotion-oriented strategies
- Uses a broad range of problem-oriented strategies
- Uses spiritual resources

READINESS FOR ENHANCED COMMUNITY COPING

(1994)

Definition *Pattern of community activities for adaptation and problem solving that is satisfactory for meeting the demands or needs of the community but can be improved for management of current and future problems/stressors*

Defining Characteristics

- One or more characteristics that indicate effective coping:
  - Active planning by community for predicted stressors
  - Active problem solving by community when faced with issues
  - Agreement that community is responsible for stress management
  - Positive communication among community members
  - Positive communication between community/aggregates and larger community
  - Programs available for recreation
  - Programs available for relaxation
  - Resources sufficient for managing stressors

Related Factors

Community has a sense of power to manage stressors

Resources available for problem solving

Social supports available

C

READINESS FOR ENHANCED FAMILY COPING
(1980)

Definition *Effective management of adaptive tasks by family member involved with the client's health challenge, who now exhibits desire and readiness for enhanced health and growth in regard to self and in relation to the client*

Defining Characteristics

- Individual expresses interest in making contact with others who have experienced a similar situation
- Family member attempts to describe growth impact of crisis

- Family member moves in direction of enriching life-style
- Family member moves in direction of health promotion
- Chooses experiences that optimize wellness

Related Factors

Adaptive tasks effectively addressed to enable goals of self-actualization to surface

Needs sufficiently gratified to enable goals of self-actualization to surface

RISK FOR SUDDEN INFANT DEATH SYNDROME
(2002, LOE 3.3)

Definition *Presence of risk factors for sudden death of an infant under 1 year of age*

Risk Factors

Modifiable
Delayed prenatal care
Infant overheating
Infant overwrapping
Infants placed to sleep in the prone position
Infants placed to sleep in the side-lying position
Lack of prenatal care
Postnatal infant smoke exposure
Prenatal infant smoke exposure
Soft underlayment (loose articles in the sleep environment)

Potentially Modifiable
Low birth weight
Prematurity
Young maternal age

Nonmodifiable
Ethnicity (e.g., African American or Native American)
Male gender
Seasonality of SIDS deaths (e.g., winter and fall months)
Infant age of 2-4 months

D

READINESS FOR ENHANCED DECISION MAKING
(2006, LOE 2.1)

Definition *A pattern of choosing courses of action that is sufficient for meeting short and long term health-related goals and can be strengthened*

Defining Characteristics

- Expresses desire to enhance decision making
- Expresses desire to enhance congruency of decisions with personal values and goals
- Expresses desire to enhance congruency of decisions with sociocultural values and goals
- Expresses desire to enhance risk benefit analysis of decisions
- Expresses desire to enhance understanding of choices for decision making
- Expresses desire to enhance understanding of the meaning of choices
- Expresses desire to enhance use of reliable evidence for decisions

References

O'Connor, A.M., Stacey, D., Entwistle, V., Llewllyn-Thomas, H., Rovner, D., Homes-Rovner, M., et al. (2005). Decision aids for people facing health treatment or screening decisions. *The Cochrane Library, Vol 3., CD-ROM Computer file.* London: BMJ Publishing Group.

Paterson, B.L., Russell, C., & Thorne, S. (2001). Critical analysis of everyday self-care decision making in chronic illness. *Journal of Advanced Nursing, 35,* 335–341.

Tunis, S.R. (2005). Perspective: A clinical research strategy to support shared decision-making. *Health Affairs, 24,* 180–184.

INEFFECTIVE DENIAL
(1988, 2006, LOE 2.1)

D

Definition *Conscious or unconscious attempt to disavow the knowledge or meaning of an event to reduce anxiety/fear, but leading to the detriment of health*

Defining Characteristics

- Delays seeking health-care attention to the detriment of health
- Displaces fear of impact of the condition
- Displaces source of symptoms to other organs
- Displays inappropriate affect
- Does not admit fear of death
- Does not admit fear of invalidism
- Does not perceive personal relevance of danger
- Does not perceive personal relevance of symptoms
- Makes dismissive comments when speaking of distressing events
- Makes dismissive gestures when speaking of distressing events
- Minimizes symptoms
- Refuses healthcare attention to the detriment of health
- Unable to admit impact of disease on life pattern
- Uses self-treatment

Related Factors

Anxiety
Fear of death
Fear of loss of autonomy
Fear of separation
Lack of competency in using effective coping mechanisms
Lack of control of life situation

Lack of emotional support from others
Overwhelming stress
Threat of inadequacy in dealing with strong emotions
Threat of unpleasant reality

continued

Ineffective Denial, *continued*

D

References

Gammon, J. (1998). Analysis of the stressful effects of hospitalisation and source isolation coping and psychological constructs. *International Journal of Nursing Practice, 4*(2), 84–96.

Mogg, K., Mathews, A., Bird, C., & MacGregor-Morris, R. (1990). Effects of stress and anxiety on the processing of threat stimuli. *Journal of Personality and Social Psychology, 59,* 1230–1237.

Sandstrom, M.J., & Cramer. P. (2003). Defense mechanisms and psychological adjustment in childhood. *Journal of Nervous and Mental Disease, 191,* 487–495.

IMPAIRED DENTITION
(1998)

D

Definition *Disruption in tooth development/eruption patterns or structural integrity of individual teeth*

Defining Characteristics

- Abraded teeth
- Absence of teeth
- Asymmetrical facial expression
- Crown caries
- Erosion of enamel
- Excessive calculus
- Excessive plaque
- Halitosis
- Incomplete eruption for age (may be primary or permanent teeth)
- Loose teeth
- Malocclusion
- Missing teeth
- Premature loss of primary teeth
- Root caries
- Tooth enamel discoloration
- Tooth fracture(s)
- Tooth misalignment
- Toothache
- Worn down teeth

Related Factors

Barriers to self-care
Bruxism
Chronic use of coffee
Chronic use of tea
Chronic use of red wine
Chronic use of tobacco
Chronic vomiting
Deficient knowledge regarding dental health
Dietary habits
Economic barriers to professional care
Excessive use of abrasive cleaning agents
Excessive intake of fluorides
Genetic predisposition
Ineffective oral hygiene
Lack of access to professional care
Nutritional deficits
Selected prescription medications
Sensitivity to cold
Sensitivity to heat

D

RISK FOR DELAYED DEVELOPMENT
(1998)

Definition *At risk for delay of 25% or more in one or more of the areas of social or self-regulatory behavior, or in cognitive, language, gross or fine motor skills*

Risk Factors

Prenatal

Endocrine disorders
Genetic disorders
Illiteracy
Inadequate nutrition
Infections
Lack of prenatal care
Late prenatal care
Maternal age <15 years
Maternal age >35 years
Poor prenatal care
Poverty
Substance abuse
Unplanned pregnancy
Unwanted pregnancy

Individual

Adopted child
Behavior disorders
Brain damage (e.g., hemorrhage in postnatal period, shaken baby, abuse, accident)
Chemotherapy
Chronic illness
Congenital disorders

Failure to thrive
Foster child
Frequent otitis media
Genetic disorders
Hearing impairment
Inadequate nutrition
Lead poisoning
Natural disasters
Positive drug screen(s)
Prematurity
Radiation therapy
Seizures
Substance abuse
Technology-dependent
Vision impairment

Environmental

Poverty
Violence

Caregiver

Abuse
Mental illness
Mental retardation
Severe learning disability

DIARRHEA
(1975, 1998)

D

Definition *Passage of loose, unformed stools*

Defining Characteristics
- Abdominal pain
- At least 3 loose liquid stools per day
- Cramping
- Hyperactive bowel sounds
- Urgency

Related Factors

Psychological

Anxiety
High stress levels

Situational

Adverse effects of medications
Alcohol abuse
Contaminants
Laxative abuse
Radiation
Toxins
Travel
Tube feedings

Physiological

Infectious processes
Inflammation
Irritation
Malabsorption
Parasites

RISK FOR COMPROMISED HUMAN DIGNITY
(2006, LOE 2.1)

D

Definition *At risk for perceived loss of respect and honor*

Risk Factors

Cultural incongruity
Disclosure of confidential information
Exposure of the body
Inadequate participation in decision making
Loss of control of body functions
Perceived dehumanizing treatment
Perceived humiliation
Perceived intrusion by clinicians
Perceived invasion of privacy
Stigmatizing label
Use of undefined medical terms

References

Shottom, L., & Seedhouse, D. (1998). Practical dignity in caring. *Nursing Ethics, 5,* 246–255.

Mairis, E. (1994). Concept clarification of professional practice-dignity. *Journal of Advanced Nursing, 19,* 924–931.

Walsh, K., & Kowanko, I. (2002). Nurses' and patients' perceptions of dignity. *International Journal of Nursing Practice, 8,* 143–151.

MORAL DISTESS
(2006, LOE 2.1)

D

Definition *Response to the inability to carry out one's chosen ethical/moral decision/action*

Defining Characteristics

- Expresses anguish (e.g., powerlessness, guilt, frustration, anxiety, self-doubt, fear) over difficulty acting on one's moral choice

Related Factors

Conflict among decision-makers

Conflicting information guiding ethical decision making

Conflicting information guiding moral decision making

Cultural conflicts

End-of-life decisions

Loss of autonomy

Physical distance of decision maker

Time constraints for decision making

Treatment decisions

References

Corley, M., Elswick, R., Gorman, M.., & Clor, T. (2001). Development and evaluation of a moral distress scale. *Journal of Advanced Nursing, 33,* 250–256.

Jameton, A. (1993). Dilemmas of moral distress: Moral responsibility and nursing practice. *AWHONN's Clinical Issues in Perinatal & Womens Health Nursing, 4,* 542–551.

Kopala, B., & Burkhart, L. (2005). Ethical dilemma and moral distress: Proposed new NANDA diagnoses. *International Journal of Nursing Terminologies and Classifications, 16,* 3–13.

D

RISK FOR DISUSE SYNDROME
(1988)

Definition   *At risk for deterioration of body systems as the result of prescribed or unavoidable musculoskeletal inactivity*

Risk Factors
Altered level of
   consciousness
Mechanical
   immobilization
Paralysis
Prescribed immobilization
Severe pain

Note.   Complications from immobility can include pressure ulcer, constipation, stasis of pulmonary secretions, thrombosis, urinary tract infection and/or retention, decreased strength or endurance, orthostatic hypotension, decreased range of joint motion, disorientation, body-image disturbance, and powerlessness.

DEFICIENT **D**IVERSIONAL ACTIVITY
(1980)

D

Definition   *Decreased stimulation from (or interest or engagement in) recreational or leisure activities*

Defining Characteristics

- Patient's statements regarding boredom (e.g., wish there was something to do, to read, etc.)
- Usual hobbies cannot be undertaken in hospital

Related Factors

Environmental lack of diversional activity

DISTURBED ENERGY FIELD
(1994, 2004, LOE 2.1)

Definition *Disruption of the flow of energy surrounding a person's being results in disharmony of the body, mind, and/or spirit*

Defining Characteristics
- Perceptions of changes in patterns of energy flow, such as
  - Movement (wave, spike, tingling, dense, flowing)
  - Sounds (tone, words)
  - Temperature change (warmth, coolness)
  - Visual changes (image, color)
  - Disruption of the field (deficit, hole, spike, bulge, obstruction, congestion, diminished flow in energy field)

Related Factors
Slowing or blocking of energy flows secondary to:

Maturational factors
  Age-related developmental crisis
  Age-related developmental difficulties

Pathophysiologic factors
  Illness
  Injury
  Pregnancy

Situational factors
  Anxiety

Fear
Grieving
Pain

Treatment-related factors
  Chemotherapy
  Immobility
  Labor and delivery
  Perioperative experience

IMPAIRED ENVIRONMENTAL INTERPRETATION SYNDROME
(1994)

Definition *Consistent lack of orientation to person, place, time, or circumstances over more than 3 to 6 months necessitating a protective environment*

Defining Characteristics

- Chronic confusional states
- Consistent disorientation
- Inability to concentrate
- Inability to follow simple directions
- Inability to reason
- Loss of occupation
- Loss of social functioning
- Slow in responding to questions

Related Factors

Dementia
Depression
Huntington's disease

F

ADULT FAILURE TO THRIVE
(1998)

Definition *Progressive functional deterioration of a physical and cognitive nature. The individual's ability to live with multisystem diseases, cope with ensuing problems, and manage his/her care are remarkably diminished.*

Defining Characteristics

- Altered mood state
- Anorexia
- Apathy
- Cognitive decline:
  - Problems with responding to environmental stimuli
  - Demonstrated difficulty in concentration
  - Demonstrated difficulty in decision making
  - Demonstrated difficulty in judgment
  - Demonstrated difficulty in memory
  - Demonstrated difficulty in reasoning
  - Decreased perception
- Consumption of minimal to no food at most meals (i.e., consumes <75% of normal requirements)
- Decreased participation in activities of daily living
- Decreased social skills
- Expresses loss of interest in pleasurable outlets
- Frequent exacerbations of chronic health problems
- Inadequate nutritional intake
- Neglect of home environment
- Neglect of financial responsibilities
- Physical decline (e.g., fatigue, dehydration, incontinence of bowel and bladder)
- Self-care deficit
- Social withdrawal
- Unintentional weight loss (e.g., 5% in 1 month, 10% in 6 months)
- Verbalizes desire for death

Related Factors

Depression

RISK FOR FALLS
(2000)

Definition   *Increased susceptibility to falling that may cause physical harm*

Risk Factors

Adults

Age 65 or over
History of falls
Lives alone
Lower limb prosthesis
Use of assistive devices (e.g., walker, cane)
Wheelchair use

Children

<2 years of age
Bed located near window
Lack of auto restraints
Lack of gate on stairs
Lack of window guard
Lack of parental supervision
Male gender when <1 year of age
Unattended infant on elevated surface (e.g., bed/changing table)

Cognitive

Diminished mental status

Environment

Cluttered environment
Dimly lit room
No antislip material in bath
No antislip material in shower
Restraints
Throw rugs
Unfamiliar room
Weather conditions (e.g., wet floors, ice)

Medications

ACE inhibitors
Alcohol use
Antianxiety agents
Antihypertensive agents
Diuretics
Hypnotics
Narcotics
Tranquilizers
Tricyclic antidepressants

Physiological

Anemias
Arthritis
Diarrhea
Decreased lower extremity strength
Difficulty with gait
Faintness when extending neck
Faintness when turning neck

continued

Risk for Falls, *continued*

Foot problems
Hearing difficulties
Impaired balance
Impaired physical
  mobility
Incontinence
Neoplasms (i.e., fatigue/
  limited mobility)
Neuropathy
Orthostatic hypotension

Postoperative conditions
Postprandial blood sugar
  changes
Presence of acute illness
Proprioceptive deficits
Sleeplessness
Urgency
Vascular disease
Visual difficulties

F

DYSFUNCTIONAL FAMILY PROCESSES: ALCOHOLISM
(1994)

Definition *Psychosocial, spiritual, and physiological functions of the family unit are chronically disorganized, which leads to conflict, denial of problems, resistance to change, ineffective problem solving, and a series of self-perpetuating crises*

F

Defining Characteristics

Behavioral

- Alcohol abuse
- Agitation
- Blaming
- Broken promises
- Chaos
- Contradictory communication
- Controlling communication
- Criticizing
- Deficient knowledge about alcoholism
- Denial of problems
- Dependency
- Difficulty having fun
- Difficulty with intimate relationships
- Difficulty with life cycle transitions
- Diminished physical contact
- Disturbances in academic performance in children
- Disturbances in concentration
- Enabling to maintain alcoholic drinking pattern
- Escalating conflict
- Failure to accomplish developmental tasks
- Family special occasions are alcohol centered
- Harsh self-judgment
- Immaturity
- Impaired communication
- Inability to accept health
- Inability to accept help
- Inability to accept a wide range of feelings
- Inability to adapt to change
- Inability to deal constructively with traumatic experiences
- Inability to express a wide range of feelings
- Inability to meet emotional needs of its members
- Inability to meet security needs of its members

continued

Dysfunctional Family Processes: Alcoholism, *continued*

- Inability to meet spiritual needs of its members
- Inability to receive help appropriately
- Inadequate understanding of alcoholism
- Inappropriate expression of anger
- Ineffective problem-solving skills
- Isolation
- Lack of dealing with conflict
- Lack of reliability
- Lying
- Manipulation
- Nicotine addiction
- Orientation toward tension relief rather than achievement of goals
- Paradoxical communication
- Power struggles
- Rationalization
- Refusal to get help
- Seeking affirmation
- Seeking approval
- Self-blaming
- Stress-related physical illnesses
- Substance abuse other than alcohol
- Unresolved grief
- Verbal abuse of children
- Verbal abuse of parent
- Verbal abuse of spouse

Feelings
- Abandonment
- Anger
- Anxiety
- Being different from other people
- Being unloved
- Confused love and pity
- Confusion
- Decreased self-esteem
- Depression
- Dissatisfaction
- Distress
- Embarrassment
- Emotional control by others
- Emotional isolation
- Failure
- Fear
- Frustration
- Guilt
- Hopelessness
- Hostility
- Hurt
- Insecurity
- Lack of identity
- Lingering resentment
- Loneliness
- Loss
- Mistrust
- Misunderstood
- Moodiness
- Powerlessness
- Rejection
- Repressed emotions

- Responsibility for alcoholic's behavior
- Supressed rage
- Shame
- Tension
- Unhappiness
- Vulnerability
- Worthlessness

Roles and Relationships

- Altered role function
- Chronic family problems
- Closed communication systems
- Deterioration in family relationships/disturbed family dynamics
- Disrupted family rituals
- Disrupted family roles
- Economic problems
- Family denial
- Family does not demonstrate respect for autonomy of its members

- Family does not demonstrate respect for individuality of its members
- Inconsistent parenting
- Ineffective spouse communication
- Intimacy dysfunction
- Lack of cohesiveness
- Lack of skills necessary for relationships
- Low perception of parental support
- Marital problems
- Neglected obligations
- Pattern of rejection
- Reduced ability of family members to relate to each other for mutual growth and maturation
- Triangulating family relationships

F

Related Factors

Abuse of alcohol
Addictive personality
Biochemical influences
Family history of alcoholism
Family history of resistance to treatment

Genetic predisposition
Inadequate coping skills
Lack of problem-solving skills

INTERRUPTED FAMILY PROCESSES
(1982, 1998)

Definition *Change in family relationships and/or functioning*

Defining Characteristics

- Changes in assigned tasks
- Changes in availability for affective responsiveness
- Changes in availability for emotional support
- Changes in communication patterns
- Changes in effectiveness in completing assigned tasks
- Changes in expressions of conflict with community resources
- Changes in expressions of isolation from community resources
- Changes in expressions of conflict within family
- Changes in intimacy
- Changes in mutual support
- Changes in patterns
- Changes in participation in problem solving
- Changes in participation in decision making
- Changes in power alliances
- Changes in rituals
- Changes in satisfaction with family
- Changes in somatic complaints
- Changes in stress-reduction behaviors

Related Factors

Developmental crises
Developmental transition
Family roles shift
Interaction with community
Modification in family finances
Modification in family
social status
Power shift of family members
Shift in health status of a family member
Situation transition
Situational crises

READINESS FOR ENHANCED FAMILY PROCESSES
(2002, LoE 2.1)

Definition *A pattern of family functioning that is sufficient to support the well-being of family members and can be strengthened*

F

Defining Characteristics

- Activities support the growth of family members
- Activities support the safety of family members
- Balance exists between autonomy and cohesiveness
- Boundaries of family members are maintained
- Communication is adequate
- Energy level of family supports activities of daily living
- Expresses willingness to enhance family dynamics
- Family adapts to change
- Family functioning meets needs of family members
- Family resilience is evident
- Family roles are appropriate for developmental stages
- Family roles are flexible for developmental stages
- Family tasks are accomplished
- Interdependent with community
- Relationships are generally positive
- Respect for family members is evident

FATIGUE
(1988, 1998)

Definition *An overwhelming sustained sense of exhaustion and decreased capacity for physical and mental work at usual level*

F

Defining Characteristics
- Compromised concentration
- Compromised libido
- Decreased performance
- Disinterest in surroundings
- Drowsy
- Feelings of guilt for not keeping up with responsibilities
- Inability to maintain usual level of physical activity
- Inability to maintain usual routines
- Inability to restore energy even after sleep
- Increase in physical complaints
- Increase in rest requirements
- Introspection
- Lack of energy
- Lethargic
- Listless
- Perceived need for additional energy to accomplish routine tasks
- Tired
- Verbalization of an unremitting lack of energy
- Verbalization of an overwhelming lack of energy

Related Factors
Psychological
  Anxiety
  Boring lifestyle
  Depression
  Stress

Physiological
  Anemia
  Disease states
  Increased physical exertion
  Malnutrition
  Poor physical condition

  Pregnancy
  Sleep deprivation

Environmental
  Humidity
  Lights
  Noise
  Temperature

Situational
  Negative life events
  Occupation

Fear
(1980, 1996, 2000)

Definition *Response to perceived threat that is consciously recognized as a danger*

Defining Characteristics

- Report of alarm
- Report of apprehension
- Report of being scared
- Report of decreased self-assurance
- Report of dread
- Report of excitement
- Report of increased tension
- Report of jitteriness
- Report of panic
- Report of terror

Cognitive

- Diminished productivity
- Diminished learning ability
- Diminished problem-solving ability
- Identifies object of fear
- Stimulus believed to be a threat

Behaviors

- Attack behaviors
- Avoidance behaviors
- Impulsiveness
- Increased alertness
- Narrowed focus on the source of the fear

Physiological

- Anorexia
- Diarrhea
- Dry mouth
- Dyspnea
- Fatigue
- Increased perspiration
- Increased pulse
- Increased respiratory rate
- Increased systolic blood pressure
- Muscle tightness
- Nausea
- Pallor
- Pupil dilation
- Vomiting

continued

Fear, *continued*

Related Factors

Innate origin (e.g., sudden noise, height, pain, loss of physical support)

Innate releasers (neurotransmitters)

Language barrier

Learned response (e.g., conditioning, modeling from or identification with others)

Phobic stimulus

Sensory impairment

Separation from support system in potentially stressful situation (e.g., hospitalization, hospital procedures)

Unfamiliarity with environmental experience(s)

F

READINESS FOR ENHANCED FLUID BALANCE
(2002, LOE 2.1)

Definition *A pattern of equilibrium between fluid volume and chemical composition of body fluids that is sufficient for meeting physical needs and can be strengthened*

F

Defining Characteristics

- Dehydration
- Expresses willingness to enhance fluid balance
- Good tissue turgor
- Intake adequate for daily needs
- Moist mucous membranes
- No evidence of edema
- No excessive thirst
- Specific gravity within normal limits
- Stable weight
- Straw-colored urine
- Urine output appropriate for intake

DEFICIENT FLUID VOLUME
(1978, 1996)

Definition   *Decreased intravascular, interstitial, and/or intracellular fluid. This refers to dehydration, water loss alone without change in sodium.*

Defining Characteristics

- Change in mental state
- Decreased blood pressure
- Decreased pulse pressure
- Decreased pulse volume
- Decreased skin turgor
- Decreased tongue turgor
- Decreased urine output
- Decreased venous filling
- Dry mucous membranes
- Dry skin
- Elevated hematocrit
- Increased body temperature
- Increased pulse rate
- Increased urine concentration
- Sudden weight loss (except in third spacing)
- Thirst
- Weakness

Related Factors

Active fluid volume loss
Failure of regulatory
   mechanisms

EXCESS FLUID VOLUME
(1982, 1996)

Definition   *Increased isotonic fluid retention*

Defining Characteristics

- Adventitious breath sounds
- Altered electrolytes
- Anascara
- Anxiety
- Azotemia
- Blood pressure changes
- Change in mental status
- Changes in respiratory pattern
- Decreased hematocrit
- Decreased hemoglobin
- Dyspnea
- Edema
- Increased central venous pressure
- Intake exceeds output
- Jugular vein distention
- Oliguria
- Orthopnea
- Pleural effusion
- Positive hepatojugular reflex
- Pulmonary artery pressure changes
- Pulmonary congestion
- Restlessness
- Specific gravity changes
- S3 heart sound
- Weight gain over short period of time

Related Factors

Compromised regulatory mechanism
Excess fluid intake
Excess sodium intake

RISK FOR DEFICIENT Fluid VOLUME
(1978)

Definition *At risk for experiencing vascular, cellular, or intracellular dehydration*

Risk Factors

Deviations affecting access of fluids

Deviations affecting intake of fluids

Deviations affecting absorption of fluids

Excessive losses through normal routes (e.g., diarrhea)

Extremes of age

Extremes of weight

Factors influencing fluid needs (e.g., hypermetabolic state)

Loss of fluid through abnormal routes (e.g., indwelling tubes)

Knowledge deficiency

Medication (e.g., diuretics)

RISK FOR IMBALANCED FLUID VOLUME
(1998)

Definition *At risk for a decrease, increase, or rapid shift from one to the other of intravascular, interstitial, and/or intracellular fluid. This refers to body fluid loss, gain, or both.*

F

Risk Factors
Scheduled for major
    invasive procedures

Note. This diagnosis will retire from the NANDA-I Taxonomy in the 2009–2010 edition unless additional work is done to bring it to a LOE of 2.1 or higher.

IMPAIRED GAS EXCHANGE
(1980, 1996, 1998)

Definition   *Excess or deficit in oxygenation and/or carbon dioxide elimination at the alveolar-capillary membrane*

Defining Characteristics

- Abnormal arterial blood gases
- Abnormal arterial pH
- Abnormal breathing (e.g., rate, rhythm, depth)
- Abnormal skin color (e.g., pale, dusky)
- Confusion
- Cyanosis (in neonates only)
- Decreased carbon dioxide
- Diaphoresis
- Dyspnea
- Headache upon awakening
- Hypercapnia
- Hypercarbia
- Hypoxemia
- Hypoxia
- Irritability
- Nasal flaring
- Restlessness
- Somnolence
- Tachycardia
- Visual disturbances

Related Factors

Alveolar-capillary
   membrane changes
Ventilation perfusion
   imbalance

RISK FOR UNSTABLE BLOOD GLUCOSE
(2006, LOE 2.1)

Definition *Risk for variation of blood glucose/sugar levels from the normal range*

Risk Factors

Deficient knowledge of diabetes management (e.g., action plan)

Developmental level

Dietary intake

Inadequate blood glucose monitoring

Lack of acceptance of diagnosis

Lack of adherence to diabetes management (e.g., action plan)

Lack of diabetes management (e.g., action plan)

Medication management

Mental health status

Physical activity level

Physical health status

Pregnancy

Rapid growth periods

Stress

Weight gain

Weight loss

References

American Diabetes Association. (2005). Standard of medical care in diabetes. *Diabetes Care, 29*, S1–S36. http://care.diabetesjournals.org/cgi/content/full/28/suppl_1/s4

Bierschbach, J., Cooper, L., & Liedl, J. (2004). Insulin pumps: What every school nurse needs to know. *Journal of School Nursing, 20*, 117–123.

U.S. Department of Health & Human Services. (2003). *Helping students with diabetes succeed: A guide for school personnel.* http://ndep.nih.gov/resources/school.htm

GRIEVING*
(1980, 1996, 2006, LOE 2.1)

Definition *A normal complex process that includes emotional, physical, spiritual, social, and intellectual responses and behaviors by which individuals, families, and communities incorporate an actual, anticipated, or perceived loss into their daily lives*

G

Defining Characteristics

- Alteration in activity level
- Alterations in immune function
- Alterations in neuroendocrine function
- Alterations in sleep patterns
- Alteration in dream patterns
- Anger
- Blame
- Detachment
- Despair
- Disorganization
- Experiencing relief
- Maintaining the connection to the deceased
- Making meaning of the loss
- Pain
- Panic behavior
- Personal growth
- Psychological distress
- Suffering

Related Factors

Anticipatory loss of significant object (e.g., possession, job, status, home, parts & processes of body)
Anticipatory loss of a significant other

Death of a significant other
Loss of significant object (e.g., possession, job, status, home, parts & processes of body)

* *Previously titled "Anticipatory Grieving"*

References

Hogan, N., Worden, J., & Schmidt, L. (2004). An empirical study of the proposed complicated grief disorder criteria. *OMEGA, 48,* 263–277.

Ott, C. (2003). The impact of complicated grief on mental and physical health at various points in the bereavement process. *Death Studies, 27,* 249–272.

Center for the Advancement of Health. (2004). Report on bereavement and grief research. *Death Studies, 28,* 498–505.

G

COMPLICATED GRIEVING*
(1980, 1986, 2004, 2006, LOE 2.1)

Definition   *A disorder that occurs after the death of a signifi-cant other, in which the experience of distress accompanying bereavement fails to follow normative expectations and mani-fests in functional impairment*

Defining Characteristics

- Decreased functioning in life roles
- Decreased sense of well-being
- Depression
- Experiencing somatic symptoms of the deceased
- Fatigue
- Grief avoidance
- Longing for the deceased
- Low levels of intimacy
- Persistent emotional distress
- Preoccupation with thoughts of the deceased
- Rumination
- Searching for the deceased
- Self-blame
- Separation distress
- Traumatic distress
- Verbalizes anxiety
- Verbalizes distressful feelings about the deceased
- Verbalizes feeling dazed
- Verbalizes feeling empty
- Verbalizes feeling in shock
- Verbalizes feeling stunned
- Verbalizes feelings of anger
- Verbalizes feelings of detachment from others
- Verbalizes feelings of disbelief
- Verbalizes feelings of mistrust
- Verbalizes lack of acceptance of the death
- Verbalizes persistent painful memories
- Verbalizes self-blame
- Yearning

* *Previously titled "Dysfunctional Grieving"*

Related Factors

Death of a significant
  other
Emotional instability
Lack of social support
Sudden death of signifi
  cant other

References

Hogan, N., Worden, J., & Schmidt, L. (2004). An empirical study of the proposed complicated grief disorder criteria. *OMEGA, 48,* 263–277.

Ott, C. (2003). The impact of complicated grief on mental and physical health at various points in the bereavement process. *Death Studies, 27,* 249–272.

Center for the Advancement of Health. (2004). Report on bereavement and grief research. *Death Studies, 28,* 498–505.

G

RISK FOR COMPLICATED GRIEVING*
(2004, 2006, LOE 2.1)

Definition   *At risk for a disorder that occurs after the death of a significant other, in which the experience of distress accompanying bereavement fails to follow normative expectations and manifests in functional impairment*

Risk Factors

Death of a significant
  other
Emotional instability
Lack of social support

References

Hogan, N., Worden, J., & Schmidt, L. (2004). An empirical study of the proposed complicated grief disorder criteria. *OMEGA, 48,* 263–277.

Ott, C. (2003). The impact of complicated grief on mental and physical health at various points in the bereavement process. *Death Studies, 27,* 249–272.

Center for the Advancement of Health. (2004). Report on bereavement and grief research. *Death Studies, 28,* 498–505.

* *Previously titled "Risk for Dysfunctional Grieving"*

DELAYED GROWTH AND DEVELOPMENT
(1986)

Definition *Deviations from age-group norms*

Defining Characteristics

- Altered physical growth
- Decreased response time
- Delay in performing skills typical of age group
- Difficulty in performing skills typical of age group
- Inability to perform self-care activities appropriate for age
- Inability to perform self-control activities appropriate for age
- Flat affect
- Listlessness

Related Factors

Effects of physical disability

Environmental deficiencies

Inadequate caretaking

Inconsistent responsiveness

Indifference

Multiple caretakers

Prescribed dependence

Separation from significant others

Stimulation deficiencies

RISK FOR DISPROPORTIONATE Gʀᴏᴡᴛʜ
(1998)

Definition *At risk for growth above the 97th percentile or below the 3rd percentile for age, crossing two percentile channels*

Risk Factors

Caregiver

Abuse
Mental illness
Mental retardation
Severe learning disability

Environmental

Deprivation
Lead poisoning
Natural disasters
Poverty
Teratogen
Violence

Individual

Anorexia
Caregiver maladaptive
    feeding behaviors
Chronic illness

Individual maladaptive
    feeding behaviors
Infection
Insatiable appetite
Prematurity
Malnutrition
Substance abuse

Prenatal

Congenital disorders
Genetic disorders
Maternal infection
Maternal nutrition
Multiple gestation
Teratogen exposure
Substance use
Substance abuse

INEFFECTIVE HEALTH MAINTENANCE
(1982)

Definition *Inability to identify, manage, and/or seek out help to maintain health*

Defining Characteristics

- Demonstrated lack of adaptive behaviors to environmental changes
- Demonstrated lack of knowledge regarding basic health practices
- Lack of expressed interest in improving health behaviors
- History of lack of health-seeking behavior
- Inability to take responsibility for meeting basic health practices
- Impairment of personal support systems

Related Factors

Cognitive impairment
Complicated grieving
Deficient communication skills
Diminished fine motor skills
Diminished gross motor skills
Inability to make appropriate judgments
Ineffective family coping
Ineffective individual coping
Insufficient resources (e.g., equipment, finances)
Lack of fine motor skills
Lack of gross motor skills
Perceptual impairment
Spiritual distress
Unachieved developmental tasks

HEALTH-SEEKING BEHAVIORS (Specify)
(1988)

Definition   *Active seeking (by a person in stable health) of ways to alter personal health habits and/or the environment in order to move toward a higher level of health*

Defining Characteristics

- Demonstrated lack of knowledge about health-promotion behaviors
- Expressed concern about current environmental conditions on health status
- Expressed desire for increased control of health practice
- Expressed desire to seek a higher level of wellness
- Observed unfamiliarity with wellness community resoucres
- Stated unfamiliarity with wellness community resources

Related Factors

To be developed

Note.   Stable health is defined as achievement of age-appropriate illness-prevention measures; client reports good or excellent health, and signs and symptoms of disease, if present, are controlled.

This diagnosis will retire from the NANDA-I Taxonomy in the 2009–2010 edition unless additional work is done to bring it to a LOE of 2.1 or higher.

IMPAIRED HOME MAINTENANCE
(1980)

Definition *Inability to independently maintain a safe growth-promoting immediate environment*

Defining Characteristics

Objective

- Disorderly surroundings
- Inappropriate household temperature
- Insufficient clothes
- Insufficient linen
- Lack of clothes
- Lack of linen
- Lack of necessary equipment
- Offensive odors
- Overtaxed family members
- Presence of vermin
- Repeated unhygienic disorders
- Repeated unhygienic infections
- Unavailable cooking equipment
- Unclean surroundings

Subjective

- Household members describe financial crises
- Household members describe outstanding debts
- Household members express difficulty in maintaining their home in a comfortable fashion
- Household members request assistance with home maintenance

Related Factors

Deficient knowledge
Disease
Inadequate support systems
Injury
Impaired functioning
Insufficient family organization
Insufficient family planning
Insufficient finances
Lack of role modeling
Unfamiliarity with neighborhood resources

READINESS FOR ENHANCED Hope
(2006, LOE 2.1)

Definition   *A pattern of expectations and desires that is suffi-cient for mobilizing energy on one's own behalf and can be strengthened*

Defining Characteristics

- Expresses desire to enhance ability to set achievable goals
- Expresses desire to enhance belief in possi-bilities
- Expresses desire to enhance congruency of expectations with desires
- Expresses desire to enhance hope

- Expresses desire to enhance interconnected-ness with others
- Expresses desire to enhance problem-solving to meet goals
- Expresses desire to enhance sense of mean-ing to life
- Expresses desire to enhance spirituality

References

Benzein, E.G. (2005). The level of and relation between hope, hope-lessness and fatigue in patients and family members in pallia-tive care. *Palliative Medicine, 19*, 234–240.

Benzein, E., & Saveman, B-L. (1998). One step towards the under-standing of hope: A concept analysis. *International Journal of Nursing Studies, 35*, 322–329.

Davis, B. (2005). Mediators of the relationship between hope and well-being in older adults. *Clinical Nursing Research, 14*, 253–272.

Hopelessness
(1986)

Definition *Subjective state in which an individual sees limited or no alternatives or personal choices available and is unable to mobilize energy on own behalf*

Defining Characteristics

- Closing eyes
- Decreased affect
- Decreased appetite
- Decreased response to stimuli
- Decreased verbalization
- Lack of initiative
- Lack of involvement in care
- Passivity
- Shrugging in response to speaker
- Sleep pattern disturbance
- Turning away from speaker
- Verbal cues (e.g., despondent content, "I can't," sighing)

Related Factors

Abandonment
Deteriorating physiological condition
Lost belief in spiritual power
Lost belief in transcendent values
Long-term stress
Prolonged activity restriction creating isolation

Hyperthermia
(1986)

Definition   *Body temperature elevated above normal range*

Defining Characteristics

- Convulsions
- Flushed skin
- Increase in body temperature above normal range
- Seizures
- Tachycardia
- Tachypnea
- Warm to touch

Related Factors

Anesthesia
Decreased perspiration
Dehydration
Exposure to hot environment
Inappropriate clothing

Increased metabolic rate
Illness
Medications
Trauma
Vigorous activity

HYPOTHERMIA
(1986, 1988)

Definition *Body temperature below normal range*

Defining Characteristics
- Body temperature below normal range
- Cool skin
- Cyanotic nail beds
- Hypertension
- Pallor
- Piloerection
- Shivering
- Slow capillary refill
- Tachycardia

H

Related Factors
Aging
Consumption of alcohol
Damage to hypothalamus
Decreased ability to shiver
Decreased metabolic rate
Evaporation from skin in cool environment
Exposure to cool environment

Illness
Inactivity
Inadequate clothing
Malnutrition
Medications
Trauma

DISTURBED PERSONAL IDENTITY
(1978)

Definition   *Inability to distinguish between self and nonself*

Defining Characteristics
- To be developed

Related Factors
To be developed

Note. This diagnosis will be retired from the NANDA-I Taxonomy with the 2009-2010 edition unless additional work is done to bring it to a LOE of 2.1.

READINESS FOR ENHANCED IMMUNIZATION STATUS
(2006, LOE 2.1)

Definition *A pattern of conforming to local, national, and/or international standards of immunization to prevent infectious disease(s) that is sufficient to protect a person, family, or community and can be strengthened*

Defining Characteristics

- Expresses desire to enhance behavior to prevent infectious disease
- Expresses desire to enhance identification of possible problems associated with immunizations
- Expresses desire to enhance identification of providers of immunizations
- Expresses desire to enhance immunization status
- Expresses desire to enhance knowledge of immunization standards
- Expresses desire to enhance record-keeping of immunizations

References

Centers for Disease Control. (2002). Recommended adult immunization schedule: United States, 2002–2003. *Mortality and Morbidity Weekly Report, 51*, 904–908.

Davis, T.C., Frederickson, D.D., Kennen, E.M., Arnold, C., Shoup, E., Sugar, M., et al. (2004). Childhood vaccine risk/benefit communication among public health clinics: A time motion study. *Public Health Nursing, 21*, 228–236.

Mell, L.K., Ogren, D.S., Davis, R.L., Mullooy, J.P., Black, S.B., Shinfield, H.R., et al. (2005). Compliance with national immunization guidelines for children younger that 2 years, 1996–1999. *Pediatrics, 115*, 461–467.

FUNCTIONAL URINARY INCONTINENCE
(1986, 1998)

Definition *Inability of usually continent person to reach toilet in time to avoid unintentional loss of urine*

Defining Characteristics

- Able to completely empty bladder
- Amount of time required to reach toilet exceeds length of time between sensing the urge to void and uncontrolled voiding
- Loss of urine before reaching toilet
- May only be incontinent in early morning
- Senses need to void

Related Factors

Altered environmental factors
Impaired cognition
Impaired vision

Neuromuscular limitations
Psychological factors
Weakened supporting pelvic structures

OVERFLOW URINARY INCONTINENCE
(2006, LOE 2.1)

Definition *Involuntary loss of urine associated with overdistention of the bladder*

Defining Characteristics
- Bladder distention
- High post-void residual volume
- Nocturia
- Observed involuntary leakage of small volumes of urine
- Reports involuntary leakage of small volumes of urine

Related Factors
Bladder outlet obstruction

Detrusor external sphincter dyssynergia

Detrusor hypocontractility

Fecal impaction

Severe pelvic prolapse

Side effects of anticholinergic medications

Side effects of calcium channel blockers

Side effects of decongestant medications

Urethral obstruction

References

Agency for Health Care Policy and Research. (1992). *Clinical practice guideline:Urinary incontinence in adults* (Pub. No. 92-0038). Rockville, MD: Author.

National Kidney and Urologic Diseases Information Clearing House. (2004). *Urinary incontinence in women.* Bethesda, MD: Author.

Walsh, P. (Ed.). (2002). *Campbell's urology* (8th ed.). Philadelphia: Saunders.

REFLEX URINARY INCONTINENCE
(1986, 1998)

Definition *Involuntary loss of urine at somewhat predictable intervals when a specific bladder volume is reached*

Defining Characteristics

- Complete emptying with lesion above pontine micturition center
- Inability to voluntarily inhibit voiding
- Inability to voluntarily initiate voiding
- Incomplete emptying with lesion above sacral micturition center
- No sensation of bladder fullness
- No sensation of urge to void
- No sensation of voiding
- Predictable pattern of voiding
- Sensation of urgency without voluntary inhibition of bladder contraction
- Sensations associated with full bladder (e.g., sweating, restlessness, abdominal discomfort)

Related Factors

Tissue damage (e.g., due to radiation cystitis, inflammatory bladder conditions, radical pelvic surgery)

Neurological impairment above level of pontine micturition center

Neurological impairment above level of sacral micturition center

STRESS URINARY INCONTINENCE
(1986, 2006, LOE 2.1)

Definition *Sudden leakage of urine with activities that increase intra-abdominal pressure*

Defining Characteristics

- Observed involuntary leakage of small amounts of urine in the absence of detrusor contraction
- Observed involuntary leakage of small amounts of urine in the absence of an over-distended bladder
- Observed involuntary leakage of small amounts of urine on exertion
- Observed involuntary leakage of small amounts of urine with sneezing, laughing, or coughing

- Reports involuntary leakage of small amounts of urine in the absence of detrusor contraction
- Reports involuntary leakage of small amounts of urine in the absence of an over-distended bladder
- Reports involuntary leakage of small amounts of urine on exertion
- Reports involuntary leakage of small amounts of urine with sneezing, laughing, or coughing

Related Factors

Degenerative changes in pelvic muscles

High intra-abdominal pressure

Intrinsic urethral sphincter deficiency

Weak pelvic muscles

References

Agency for Health Care Policy and Research. (1992). *Clinical practice guideline: Urinary incontinence in adults* (AHCPR Pub. No. 92-0038). Rockville, MD: Author.

National Kidney and Urologic Diseases Information Clearing House. (2004). *Urinary incontinence in women.* Retrieved January 27, 2005 from *http://kidney.niddk.nih.gov/kudiseases/pubs/uiwomen/index.htm.*

NIH consensus statements. (1988). *Urinary incontinence in adults.* Retrieved January 27, 2005 from *http://consensus.nih.gov/cons/071/071_statement.htm.*

TOTAL URINARY INCONTINENCE
(1986)

Definition   *Continuous and unpredictable loss of urine*

Defining Characteristics

- Constant flow of urine at unpredictable times without uninhibited bladder contractions/spasm or distention
- Lack of bladder filling
- Lack of perineal filling
- Nocturia
- Unawareness of incontinence
- Unsuccessful incontinence refractory treatments

Related Factors

Anatomic (fistula)

Disease affecting spinal cord nerves

Independent contraction of detrusor reflex

Neurological dysfunction

Neuropathy preventing transmission of reflex indicating bladder fullness

Trauma affecting spinal cord nerves

Note.   This diagnosis will retire from the NANDA-I Taxonomy in the 2009–2010 edition unless additional work is done to bring it to a LOE of 2.1 or higher.

URGE URINARY INCONTINENCE
(1986, 2006, LOE 2.1)

Definition   *Involuntary passage of urine occurring soon after a strong sense of urgency to void*

Defining Characteristics

- Observed inability to reach toilet in time to avoid urine loss
- Reports urinary urgency
- Reports involuntary loss of urine with bladder contractions / spasms
- Reports inability to reach toilet in time to avoid urine loss

Related Factors

Alcohol intake
Atrophic urethritis
Atrophic vaginitis
Bladder infection
Caffeine intake
Decreased bladder capacity

Detrusor hyperactivity with impaired bladder contractility
Fecal impaction
Use of diuretics

References

Agency for Health Care Policy and Research (AHCPR). (1992). *Clinical practice guideline: Urinary incontinence in adults* (AHCPR Pub. No. 92-0038). Rockville, MD: Author.

National Kidney and Urologic Diseases Information Clearing House (NIDDK). (2004). *Urinary incontinence in women.* Retrieved January 27, 2005 from *http://kidney.niddk.nih.gov/kudiseases/pubs/uiwomen/index.htm.*

NIH consensus statements. (1988). *Urinary incontinence in adults.* Retrieved January 27, 2005 from *http://consensus.nih.gov/cons/071/071_statement.htm.*

RISK FOR URGE URINARY INCONTINENCE
(1998)

Definition *At risk for involuntary loss of urine associated with a sudden, strong sensation or urinary urgency*

Risk Factors

Effects of alcohol
Effects of caffeine
Effects of medications
Detrusor hyperreflexia
(e.g., from cystitis, urethritis, tumors, renal
calculi, central nervous
system disorders above
pontine micturition
center)

Impaired bladder
contractility
Involuntary sphincter
relaxation
Ineffective toileting
habits
Small bladder capacity

DISORGANIZED INFANT BEHAVIOR
(1994, 1998)

Definition *Disintegrated physiological and neurobehavioral responses of infant to the environment*

Defining Characteristics

Attention-Interaction System

- Abnormal response to sensory stimuli (e.g., difficult to soothe, inability to sustain alert status)

Motor System

- Altered primitive reflexes
- Changes to motor tone
- Finger splaying
- Fisting
- Hands to face
- Hyperextension of extremities
- Jittery
- Startles
- Tremors
- Twitches
- Uncoordinated movement

Physiological

- Arrhythmias
- Bradycardia
- Desaturation
- Feeding intolerances

- Skin color changes
- Tachycardia
- Time-out signals (e.g., gaze, grasp, hiccough, cough, sneeze, sigh, slack jaw, open mouth, tongue thrust)

Regulatory Problems

- Inability to inhibit startle
- Irritability

State-Organization System

- Active-awake (fussy, worried gaze)
- Diffuse sleep
- Irritable crying
- State-oscillation
- Quiet-awake (staring, gaze aversion)

continued

Disorganized Infant Behavior, *continued*

Related Factors

Caregiver

Cue knowledge deficit
Cue misreading
Environmental stimulation contribution

Environmental

Lack of containment within environment
Physical environment inappropriateness
Sensory deprivation
Sensory inappropriateness
Sensory overstimulation

Individual

Gestational age
Illness
Immature neurological system
Postconceptual age

Postnatal

Feeding intolerance
Invasive procedures
Malnutrition
Motor problems
Oral problems
Pain
Prematurity

Prenatal

Congenital disorders
Genetic disorders
Teratogenic exposure

RISK FOR DISORGANIZED INFANT BEHAVIOR
(1994)

Definition *Risk for alteration in integrating and modulation of the physiological and behavioral systems of functioning (i.e., autonomic, motor, state, organizational, self-regulatory, and attentional-interactional systems)*

Risk Factors

Environmental overstim-
  ulation
Invasive procedures
Lack of containment
  within environment
Motor problems
Oral problems
Pain
Painful procedures
Prematurity

READINESS FOR ENHANCED ORGANIZED INFANT BEHAVIOR
(1994)

Definition *A pattern of modulation of the physiologic and behavioral systems of functioning (i.e., autonomic, motor, state-organizational, self-regulatory, and attentional-interactional systems) in an infant that is satisfactory but that can be improved*

Defining Characteristics
- Definite sleep-wake states
- Response to stimuli (e.g., visual, auditory)
- Stable physiologic measures
- Use of some self-regulatory behaviors

Related Factors
Pain
Prematurity

INEFFECTIVE INFANT FEEDING PATTERN
(1992, 2006, LOE 2.1)

Definition *Impaired ability of an infant to suck or coordinate the suck/swallow response resulting in inadequate oral nutrition for metabolic needs*

Defining Characteristics

- Inability to coordinate sucking, swallowing, and breathing
- Inability to initiate an effective suck
- Inability to sustain an effective suck

Related Factors

Anatomic abnormality
Neurological delay
Neurological impairment
Oral hypersensitivity
Prematurity
Prolonged NPO status

References

Hazinski, M.F. (1992). *Nursing care of the critically ill child.* St. Louis, MO: Mosby.

Shaker, C.S. (1991). Nipple feeding premature infants: A different perspective. *Neonatal Network: The Journal of Neonatal Nursing,* *8*(5), 9–17.

VandenBerg, K. (1990). Nippling management of the sick neonate in the NICU: The disorganized feeder. *Neonatal Network: The Journal of Neonatal Nursing,* 9(1), 9–16.

RISK FOR INFECTION
(1986)

Definition *At increased risk for being invaded by pathogenic organisms*

Risk Factors

Chronic disease

Inadequate acquired immunity

Inadequate primary defenses (broken skin, traumatized tissue, decrease in ciliary action, stasis of body fluids, change in pH secretions, altered peristalsis)

Inadequate secondary defenses (decreased hemoglobin, leukopenia, suppressed inflammatory response)

Increased environmental exposure to pathogens

Immunosuppression

Invasive procedures

Insufficient knowledge to avoid exposure to pathogens

Malnutrition

Pharmaceutical agents (e.g., immunosuppressants)

Rupture of amniotic membranes

Trauma

Tissue destruction

RISK FOR INJURY
(1978)

Definition *At risk of injury as a result of environmental conditions interacting with the individual's adaptive and defensive resources*

Risk Factors

External

Biological (e.g., immunization level of community, microorganism)

Chemical (e.g., poisons, pollutants, drugs, pharmaceutical agents, alcohol, nicotine, preservatives, cosmetics, dyes)

Human (e.g., nosocomial agents; staffing patterns; cognitive, affective, psychomotor factors)

Mode of transport

Nutritional (e.g., vitamins, food types)

Physical (e.g., design, structure, and arrangement of community, building, and/or equipment)

Internal

Abnormal blood profile (e.g., leukocytosis/leukopenia, altered clotting factors, thrombocytopenia, sickle cell, thalassemia, decreased hemoglobin)

Biochemical dysfunction

Developmental age (physiological, psychosocial)

Effector dysfunction

Immune-autoimmune dysfunction

Integrative dysfunction

Malnutrition

Physical (e.g., broken skin, altered mobility)

Psychological (affective orientation)

Sensory dysfunction

Tissue hypoxia

RISK FOR PERIOPERATIVE-POSITIONING INJURY
(1994, 2006, LOE 2.1)

Definition *At risk for inadvertent anatomical and physical changes as a result of posture or equipment used during an invasive/surgical procedure*

Risk Factors

Disorientation
Edema
Emaciation
Immobilization
Muscle weakness
Obesity
Sensory/perceptual dis-
   turbances due to anes-
   thesia

References

Ali, A., Breslin, D., Hardman, H., & Martin, G. (2003). Unusual presentation and complication of the prone position for spinal surgery. *Journal of Clinical Anesthesia, 15,* 471–473.

Fritzlen, T., Kremer, M., & Biddle, C. (2003). The AANA Foundation Closed Malpractice Claims Study on nerve injuries during anesthesia care. *AANA Journal, 71,* 347–352.

Litwiller, J., Wells, R. Jr, Halliwill, J., Carmichael, S., & Warner, M. (2004). Effect of lithotomy positions on strain of the obturator and lateral femoral cutaneous nerves. *Clinical Anatomy, 17,* 45–49.

INSOMNIA*
(2006, LOE 2.1)

Definition *A disruption in amount and quality of sleep that impairs functioning*

Defining Characteristics

- Observed changes in affect
- Observed lack of energy
- Increased work/school absenteeism
- Patient reports changes in mood
- Patient reports decreased health status
- Patient reports decreased quality of life
- Patient reports difficulty concentrating
- Patient reports difficulty falling asleep
- Patient reports difficulty staying asleep
- Patient reports dissatisfaction with sleep (current)
- Patient reports increased accidents
- Patient reports lack of energy
- Patient reports non-restorative sleep
- Patient reports sleep disturbances that produce next-day consequences
- Patient reports waking up too early

Related Factors

Activity pattern (e.g., timing, amount)
Anxiety
Depression
Environmental factors (e.g., ambient noise, daylight/darkness exposure, ambient temperature/humidity, unfamiliar setting)
Fear
Gender-related hormonal shifts
Grief
Inadequate sleep hygiene (current)
Intake of stimulants
Intake of alcohol

continued

* Previously titled "Disturbed Sleep Pattern"

Insomnia, *continued*

Impairment of normal sleep pattern (e.g. travel, shift work, parental responsibilities, interruptions for interventions)

Medications

Physical discomfort (e.g., body temperature, pain, shortness of breath, cough, gastroesophageal reflux, nausea, incontinence/urgency)

Stress (e.g., ruminative pre-sleep pattern)

References

Linton, S., & Bryngelsson, I. (2000). Insomnia and its relationship to work and health in a working-age population. *Journal of Occupational Rehabilitation, 10,* 169–183.

Sateia, M., & Nowell, P. (2004). Insomnia. *Lancet, 364,* 1959–1973.

Walsh, J. (1999). Insomnia: Prevalence and clinical and public health considerations. *Family Practice Recertification, 21*(10), 4–11.

DECREASED INTRACRANIAL ADAPTIVE CAPACITY
(1994)

Definition *Intracranial fluid dynamic mechanisms that normally compensate for increases in intracranial volumes are compromised, resulting in repeated disproportionate increases in intracranial pressure (ICP) in response to a variety of noxious and nonnoxious stimuli*

Defining Characteristics
- Baseline ICP ≤ 10 mm Hg
- Disproportionate increase in ICP following stimulus
- Elevated P_2 ICP wave form
- Repeated increases of >10 mm Hg for more than 5 minutes following any of a variety of external stimuli
- Volume pressure response test variation (volume-pressure ratio 2, pressure-volume index <10)
- Wide amplitude ICP wave form

Related Factors
Brain injuries
Decreased cerebral perfusion ≤ 50–60 mm Hg
Sustained increase in ICP = 10–15 mm Hg
Systemic hypotension with intracranial hypertension

DEFICIENT **K**NOWLEDGE (Specify)
(1980)

Definition   *Absence or deficiency of cognitive information related to a specific topic*

Defining Characteristics

- Exaggerated behaviors
- Inaccurate follow through of instruction
- Inaccurate performance of test
- Inappropriate behaviors (e.g., hysterical, hostile, agitated, apathetic)
- Verbalization of the problem

Related Factors

Cognitive limitation
Information misinterpretation
Lack of exposure
Lack of interest in learning
Lack of recall
Unfamiliarity with information resources

READINESS FOR ENHANCED
Knowledge
(2002, LOE 2.1)

Definition *The presence or acquisition of cognitive information related to a specific topic is sufficient for meeting health-related goals and can be strengthened*

Defining Characteristics

- Behaviors congruent with expressed knowledge
- Explains knowledge of the topic
- Expresses an interest in learning
- Describes previous experiences pertaining to the topic

SEDENTARY LIFESTYLE
(2004, LOE 2.1)

Definition *Reports a habit of life that is characterized by a low physical activity level*

Defining Characteristics

- Chooses a daily routine lacking physical exercise
- Demonstrates physical deconditioning
- Verbalizes preference for activities low in physical activity

Risk Factors

Deficient knowledge of health benefits of physical exercise

Lack of interest

Lack of motivation

Lack of resources (time, money, companionship, facilities)

Lack of training for accomplishment of physical exercise

RISK FOR IMPAIRED LIVER FUNCTION
(2006, LOE 2.1)

Definition   *At risk for liver dysfunction*

Risk Factors

- Hepatotoxic medications (e.g., acetaminophen, statins)
- HIV co-infection
- Substance abuse (e.g., alcohol, cocaine)
- Viral infection (e.g., hepatitis A, hepatitis B, hepatitis C, Epstein-Barr)

References

AASLD Practice Guideline. (2004). *Diagnosis, management, and treatment of hepatitis C.* Alexandria, VA: American Association for the Study of Liver Diseases.

Hoofnagle, J.H., & Seeff, L.B. (2002). National Institute of Health consensus development conference: Management of hepatitis C. *Hepatology* (Suppl. 1), 1-20.

Palmer, M. (2000). *Hepatitis liver disease: What you need to know.* Garden City Park, NY, Avery Publishing Group.

L

RISK FOR LONELINESS
(1994, 2006, LOE 2.1)

Definition   *At risk for experiencing discomfort associated with a desire or need for more contact with others*

Risk Factors
Affectional deprivation
Cathectic deprivation
Physical isolation
Social isolation

References

Leiderman, P.H. (1969). Loneliness: A psychodynamic interpretation. In E.S. Scheidman & M.J. Ortega (Eds.), *Aspects of depression: International psychiatry clinics, 6*, 155–174. Boston: Little, Brown.
Lien-Gieschen, T. (1993). Validation of social isolation related to maturational age: Elderly. *Nursing Diagnosis, 4*(1), 37–44.
Warren, B.J. (1993). Explaining social isolation through concept analysis. *Archives of Psychiatric Nursing, 7*, 270–276.

IMPAIRED MEMORY
(1994)

Definition *Inability to remember or recall bits of information or behavioral skills*

Defining Characteristics

- Experience of forgetting
- Forgets to perform a behavior at a scheduled time
- Inability to determine if a behavior was performed
- Inability to learn new information
- Inability to learn new skills
- Inability to perform a previously learned skill
- Inability to recall events
- Inability to recall factual information
- Inability to retain new information
- Inability to retain new skills

Related Factors

Anemia
Decreased cardiac output
Excessive environmental disturbances
Fluid and electrolyte imbalance
Hypoxia
Neurological disturbances

IMPAIRED BED MOBILITY
(1998, 2006, LOE 2.1)

Definition *Limitation of independent movement from one bed position to another*

Defining Characteristics

- Impaired ability to move from supine to sitting
- Impaired ability to move from sitting to supine
- Impaired ability to move from supine to prone
- Impaired ability to move from prone to supine
- Impaired ability to move from supine to long sitting
- Impaired ability to move from long sitting to supine
- Impaired ability to "scoot" or reposition self in bed
- Impaired ability to turn from side to side

Related Factors

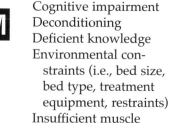

Cognitive impairment
Deconditioning
Deficient knowledge
Environmental constraints (i.e., bed size, bed type, treatment equipment, restraints)
Insufficient muscle strength

Musculoskeletal impairment
Neuromuscular impairment
Obesity
Pain
Sedating medications

Note. Specify level of independence using a standardized funtional scale.

References

Brouwer, K., Nysseknabm, J., & Culham E. (2004). Physical function and health status among seniors with and without fear of falling. *Gerontology, 50,* 15–141.

Lewis, C.L., Moutoux, M., Slaughter, M., & Bailey, S.P. (2004). Characteristics of individuals who fell while receiving home health services. *Physical Therapy,* 84(1), 23–32.

Tinetti., M.E., & Ginter, S.F. (1988). Identifying mobility dysfunction in elderly persons. *Journal of American Medical Association, 259,* 1190–1193.

IMPAIRED PHYSICAL MOBILITY
(1973, 1998)

Definition *Limitation in independent, purposeful physical movement of the body or of one or more extremities*

Defining Characteristics

- Decreased reaction time
- Difficulty turning
- Engages in substitutions for movement (e.g., increased attention to other's activity, controlling behavior, focus on pre-illness disability/activity)
- Exertional dyspnea
- Gait changes
- Jerky movements
- Limited ability to perform gross motor skills
- Limited ability to perform fine motor skills
- Limited range of motion
- Movement-induced tremor
- Postural instability
- Slowed movement
- Uncoordinated movements

Related Factors

Activity intolerance
Altered cellular metabolism
Anxiety
Body mass index above 75th age-appropriate percentile
Cognitive impairment
Contractures
Cultural beliefs regarding age-appropriate activity
Deconditioning
Decreased endurance

Depressive mood state
Decreased muscle control
Decreased muscle mass
Decreased muscle strength
Deficient knowledge regarding value of physical activity
Developmental delay
Discomfort
Disuse
Joint stiffness

Note. Specify level of independence using a standardized functional scale.

Lack of environmental supports (e.g., physical or social)

Limited cardiovascular endurance

Loss of integrity of bone structures

Malnutrition

Medications

Musculoskeletal impairment

Neuromuscular impairment

Pain

Prescribed movement restrictions

Reluctance to initiate movement

Sedentary lifestyle

Sensoriperceptual impairments

IMPAIRED WHEELCHAIR MOBILITY
(1998, 2006, LOE 2.1)

Definition *Limitation of independent operation of wheelchair within environment*

Defining Characteristics

- Impaired ability to operate manual wheelchair on curbs
- Impaired ability to operate power wheelchair on curbs
- Impaired ability to operate manual wheelchair on even surface
- Impaired ability to operate power wheelchair on even surface
- Impaired ability to operate manual wheelchair on uneven surface
- Impaired ability to operate power wheelchair on uneven surface
- Impaired ability to operate manual wheelchair on an incline
- Impaired ability to operate power wheelchair on an incline
- Impaired ability to operate manual wheelchair on a decline
- Impaired ability to operate power wheelchair on a decline

Related Factors

Cognitive impairment
Deconditioning
Deficient knowledge
Depressed mood
Environmental constraints (e.g., stairs, inclines, uneven surfaces, unsafe obstacles, distances, lack of assistive devices or person, wheelchair type)
Impaired vision
Insufficient muscle strength
Limited endurance
Musculoskeletal impairment (e.g., contractures)

Note. Specify level of independence using a standardized functional scale.

Neuromuscular impair-
ment
Obesity
Pain

References

Brouwer, K., Nysseknabm, J., & Culham E. (2004). Physical function and health status among seniors with and without fear of falling. *Gerontology, 50,* 15–141.

Lewis, C.L., Moutoux, M., Slaughter, M., & Bailey, S.P. (2004). Characteristics of individuals who fell while receiving home health services. *Physical Therapy, 84*(1), 23–32.

Tinetti., M.E., & Ginter, S.F. (1988). Identifying mobility dysfunction in elderly persons. *Journal of the American Medical Association, 259,* 1190–1193

NAUSEA

(1998, 2002, LOE 2.1)

Definition *A subjective unpleasant, wavelike sensation in the back of the throat, epigastrium, or abdomen that may lead to the urge or need to vomit*

Defining Characteristics

- Aversion toward food
- Gagging sensation
- Increased salivation
- Increased swallowing
- Report of nausea
- Sour taste in mouth

Related Factors

Biophysical

Biochemical disorders (e.g., uremia, diabetic ketoacidosis, pregnancy)
Esophageal disease
Gastric distention
Gastric irritation
Increased intracranial pressure
Intra-abdominal tumors
Labyrinthitis
Liver capsule stretch
Localized tumors (e.g., acoustic neuroma, primary or secondary brain tumors, bone metastases at base of skull)
Meningitis
Ménière's disease
Motion sickness
Pain
Pancreatic disease
Splenetic capsule stretch

Toxins (e.g., tumor-pro-
duced peptides, abnor-
mal metabolites due to
cancer)

Situational

Anxiety
Fear
Noxious odors
Noxious taste
Pain
Psychological factors
Unpleasant visual stim-
ulation

Treatment

Gastric distention
Gastric irritation
Pharmaceuticals

N

UNILATERAL NEGLECT
(1986, 2006, LOE 2.1)

Definition *Impairment in sensory and motor response, mental representation, and spatial attention of the body and the corresponding environment characterized by inattention to one side and overattention to the opposite side. Left side neglect is more severe and persistent than right side neglect.*

Defining Characteristics

- Appears unaware of positioning of neglected limb
- Difficulty remembering details of internally represented familiar scenes that are on the neglected side
- Displacement of sounds to the non-neglected side
- Distortion of drawing on the half of the page on the neglected side
- Failure to cancel lines on the half of the page on the neglected side
- Failure to eat food from portion of the plate on the neglected side
- Failure to dress neglected side
- Failure to groom neglected side
- Failure to move eyes in the neglected hemispace despite being aware of a stimulus in that space
- Failure to move head in the neglected hemispace despite being aware of a stimulus in that space
- Failure to move limbs in the neglected hemispace despite being aware of a stimulus in that space
- Failure to move trunk in the neglected hemispace despite being aware of a stimulus in that space
- Failure to notice people approaching from the neglected side
- Lack of safety precautions with regard to the neglected side
- Marked deviation* of the eyes to the non-neglected side to stimuli and activities on that side

*As if drawn magnetically to stimuli and activities on that side

- Marked deviation* of the head to the non-neglected side to stimuli and activities on that side
- Marked deviation* of the trunk to the non-neglected side to stimuli and activities on that side
- Omission of drawing on the half of the page on the neglected side
- Perseveration of visual motor tasks on non-neglected side
- Substitution of letters to form alternative words that are similar to the original in length when reading
- Transfer of pain sensation to the non-neglected side
- Use of only vertical half of page when writing

Related Factors

Brain injury from cerebrovascular problems
Brain injury from neurological illness
Brain injury from trauma
Brain injury from tumor

Left hemiplegia from CVA of the right hemisphere
Hemianopsia

N

References

Rusconi, M.L., Maravita, A., Bottini, G., & Vallar, G. (2002). Is the intact side really intact? Perseverative responses in patients with unilateral neglect: A productive manifestation. *Neuropsychologia*, 40, 594–604.

Swan, L. (2001). Unilateral spatial neglect. *Physical Therapy, 81,* 1572–1580.

Weitzel, E.A. (2001); Unilateral neglect. In M. Maas, K. Buckwalter, M. Hardy, T. Tripp-Reimer, M. Titler, & J. Specht (Eds.), *Nursing care of older adults: Diagnosis, outcomes, and interventions* (pp. 492–502): St. Louis: Mosby, Inc.

*As if drawn magnetically to stimuli and activities on that side

NONCOMPLIANCE
(1973, 1996, 1998)

Definition *Behavior of person and/or caregiver that fails to coincide with a health-promoting or therapeutic plan agreed on by the person (and/or family and/or community) and health-care professional. In the presence of an agreed-on, health-promoting or therapeutic plan, person's or caregiver's behavior is fully or partially nonadherent and may lead to clinically ineffective or partially ineffective outcomes.*

Defining Characteristics

- Behavior indicative of failure to adhere
- Evidence of development of complications
- Evidence of exacerbation of symptoms
- Failure to keep appointments
- Failure to progress
- Objective tests (e.g., physiological measures, detection of physiologic markers)

Related Factors

Health System

Access to care
Client/provider relationships
Communication skills of the provider
Convenience of care
Credibility of provider
Individual health coverage
Provider continuity
Provider regular follow-up
Provider reimbursement
Satisfaction with care
Teaching skills of the provider

Healthcare Plan

Complexity
Cost
Duration
Financial flexibility of plan
Intensity

Individual

Cultural influences
Developmental abilities
Health beliefs
Individual's value system

Knowledge relevant to
  the regimen behavior
Motivational forces
Personal abilities
Significant others
Skill relevant to the regimen behavior
Spiritual values

Network
  Involvement of members
    in health plan
  Perceived beliefs of significant others
  Social value regarding plan

N

IMBALANCED NUTRITION: LESS THAN BODY REQUIREMENTS
(1975, 2000)

Definition   *Intake of nutrients insufficient to meet metabolic needs*

Defining Characteristics

- Abdominal cramping
- Abdominal pain
- Aversion to eating
- Body weight 20% or more under ideal
- Capillary fragility
- Diarrhea
- Excessive loss of hair
- Hyperactive bowel sounds
- Lack of food
- Lack of information
- Lack of interest in food
- Loss of weight with adequate food intake
- Misconceptions
- Misinformation
- Pale mucous membranes
- Perceived inability to ingest food
- Poor muscle tone
- Reported altered taste sensation
- Reported food intake less than RDA (recommended daily allowance)
- Satiety immediately after ingesting food
- Sore buccal cavity
- Steatorrhea
- Weakness of muscles required for swallowing or mastication

Related Factors

Biological factors
Economic factors
Inability to absorb nutrients
Inability to digest food
Inability to ingest food
Psychological factors

IMBALANCED NUTRITION: MORE THAN BODY REQUIREMENTS
(1975, 2000)

Definition *Intake of nutrients that exceeds metabolic needs*

Defining Characteristics

- Concentrating food intake at the end of the day
- Dysfunctional eating pattern (e.g., pairing food with other activities)
- Eating in response to external cues (e.g., time of day, social situation)
- Eating in response to internal cues other than hunger (e.g., anxiety)
- Sedentary activity level
- Triceps skin fold >25 mm in women, >15 mm in men
- Weight 20% over ideal for height and frame

Related Factors

Excessive intake in relation to metabolic need

N

READINESS FOR ENHANCED NUTRITION
(2002, LOE 2.1)

Definition *A pattern of nutrient intake that is sufficient for meeting metabolic needs and can be strengthened*

Defining Characteristics

- Attitude toward drinking is congruent with health goals
- Attitude toward eating is congruent with health goals
- Consumes adequate fluid
- Consumes adequate food
- Eats regularly
- Expresses knowledge of healthy fluid choices
- Expresses knowledge of healthy food choices
- Expresses willingness to enhance nutrition
- Follows an appropriate standard for intake (e.g., the food pyramid or America Diabetic Association guidelines)
- Safe preparation for fluids
- Safe preparation for food
- Safe storage for food and fluids

N

RISK FOR IMBALANCED NUTRITION: MORE THAN BODY REQUIREMENTS
(1980, 2000)

Definition *At risk for an intake of nutrients that exceeds metabolic needs*

Risk Factors

Concentrating food intake at end of day

Dysfunctional eating patterns

Eating in response to external cues (e.g., time of day, social situation)

Eating in response to internal cues other than hunger (e.g., anxiety)

Higher baseline weight at beginning of each pregnancy

Observed use of food as comfort measure

Observed use of food as reward

Pairing food with other activities

Parental obesity

Rapid transition across growth percentiles in children

Reported use of solid food as major food source before 5 months of age

IMPAIRED ORAL MUCOUS MEMBRANE
(1982, 1998)

Definition *Disruption of the lips and/or soft tissue of the oral cavity*

Defining Characteristics

- Bleeding
- Cheilitis
- Coated tongue
- Desquamation
- Difficult speech
- Difficulty eating
- Difficulty swallowing
- Diminished taste
- Edema
- Enlarged tonsils
- Fissures
- Geographic tongue
- Gingival hyperplasia
- Gingival pallor
- Gingival recession
- Halitosis
- Hyperemia
- Macroplasia
- Mucosal denudation
- Mucosal pallor
- Nodules
- Oral discomfort
- Oral lesions
- Oral pain
- Oral ulcers
- Papules
- Pocketing deeper than 4 mm
- Presence of pathogens
- Purulent drainage
- Purulent exudates
- Red or bluish masses (e.g., hemangiomas)
- Reports bad taste in mouth
- Smooth atrophic tongue
- Spongy patches
- Stomatitis
- Vesicles
- White, curd-like exudate
- White patches/plaques
- Xerostomia

Related Factors

Barriers to oral self-care
Barriers to professional
  care
Chemotherapy
Chemical irritants (e.g.,
  alcohol, tobacco, acidic
  foods, drugs, regular
  use of inhalers or other
  noxious agents)
Cleft lip
Cleft palate
Decreased platelets
Decreased salivation
Deficient knowledge of
  appropriate oral
  hygiene
Dehydration
Depression
Diminished hormone lev-
  els (women)

Ineffective oral hygiene
Infection
Immunocompromised
Immunosuppression
Loss of supportive struc-
  tures
Malnutrition
Mechanical factors (e.g.,
  ill-fitting dentures,
  braces, tubes [endotra-
  cheal/nasogastric],
  surgery in oral cavity)
Medication side effects
Mouth breathing
NPO for more than 24
  hours
Radiation therapy
Stress
Trauma

ACUTE PAIN
(1996)

Definition *Unpleasant sensory and emotional experience arising from actual or potential tissue damage or described in terms of such damage (International Association for the Study of Pain); sudden or slow onset of any intensity from mild to severe with an anticipated or predictable end and a duration of less than 6 months*

Defining Characteristics

- Change in muscle tone (may span from listless to rigid)
- Changes in appetite
- Changes in blood pressure
- Changes in heart rate
- Changes in respiratory rate
- Coded report
- Diaphoresis
- Distraction behavior (e.g., pacing, seeking out other people and/or activities, repetitive activities)
- Expressive behavior (e.g., restlessness, moaning, crying, vigilance, irritability, sighing)
- Facial mask
- Guarding behavior
- Narrowed focus (altered time perception, impaired thought processes, reduced interaction with people and environment)
- Observed evidence of pain
- Positioning to avoid pain
- Protective gestures
- Pupillary dilation
- Self-focus
- Sleep disturbance (eyes lack luster, beaten look, fixed or scattered movement, grimace)
- Verbal report of pain

Related Factors

Injury agents (biological, chemical, physical, psychological)

CHRONIC Pain
(1986, 1996)

Definition *Unpleasant sensory and emotional experience arising from actual or potential tissue damage or described in terms of such damage (International Association for the Study of Pain); sudden or slow onset of any intensity from mild to severe, constant or recurring without an anticipated or predictable end and a duration of greater than 6 months*

Defining Characteristics

- Altered ability to continue previous activities
- Anorexia
- Atrophy of involved muscle group
- Changes in sleep pattern
- Coded report
- Depression
- Facial mask
- Fatigue
- Fear of reinjury
- Guarding behavior
- Irritability
- Observed protective behavior,
- Reduced interaction with people
- Restlessness
- Self-focusing
- Sympathetic mediated responses (e.g., temperature, cold, changes of body position, hypersensitivity)
- Verbal report of pain

Related Factors

Chronic physical disability
Chronic psychosocial disability

READINESS FOR ENHANCED PARENTING
(2002, LOE 2.1)

Definition *A pattern of providing an environment for children or other dependent person(s) that is sufficient to nurture growth and development and can be strengthened*

Defining Characteristics
- Children or other dependent person(s) express(es) satisfaction with home environment
- Emotional support of children
- Evidence of attachment
- Exhibits realistic expectations of children
- Expresses willingness to enhance parenting
- Needs of children are met (e.g., physical and emotional)

P

IMPAIRED PARENTING
(1978, 1998)

Definition *Inability of the primary caretaker to create, maintain, or regain an environment that promotes the optimum growth and development of the child*

Defining Characteristics

Infant or Child

- Behavioral disorders
- Failure to thrive
- Frequent accidents
- Frequent illness
- Incidence of abuse
- Incidence of trauma (e.g., physical and psychological)
- Lack of attachment
- Lack of separation anxiety
- Poor academic performance
- Poor cognitive development
- Poor social competence
- Runaway

Parental

- Abandonment
- Child abuse
- Child neglect
- Frequently punitive
- Hostility to child
- Inadequate attachment
- Inadequate child health maintenance
- Inappropriate caretaking skills

- Inappropriate stimulation (e.g., visual, tactile, auditory)
- Inappropriate child care arrangements
- Inconsistent behavior management
- Inconsistent care
- Inflexibility in meeting needs of child
- Little cuddling
- Maternal-child interaction deficit
- Negative statements about child
- Poor parent-child interaction
- Rejection of child
- Statements of inability to meet child's needs
- Unsafe home environment
- Verbalization of inability to control child
- Verbalization of frustration
- Verbalization of role inadequacy

continued

P

Impaired Parenting, *continued*

Related Factors
Infant or Child

Altered perceptual abilities
Attention deficit hyperactivity disorder
Developmental delay
Difficult temperament
Handicapping condition
Illness
Multiple births
Not desired gender
Premature birth
Separation from parent
Temperamental conflicts with parental expectations

Knowledge

Deficient knowledge about child development
Deficient knowledge about child health maintenance
Deficient knowledge about parenting skills
Inability to respond to infant cues
Lack of cognitive readiness for parenthood
Lack of education
Limited cognitive functioning
Poor communication skills

Preference for physical punishment
Unrealistic expectations

Physiological

Physical illness

Psychological

Closely spaced pregnancies
Depression
Difficult birthing process
Disability
High number of pregnancies
History of mental illness
History of substance abuse
Lack of prenatal care
Sleep deprivation
Sleep disruption
Young parental age

Social

Change in family unit
Chronic low self-esteem
Father of child not involved
Financial difficulties
History of being abused
History of being abusive
Inability to put child's needs before own
Inadequate child care arrangements

Job problems
Lack of family cohesiveness
Lack of parental role model
Lack of resources
Lack of social support networks
Lack of transportation
Lack of valuing of parenthood
Legal difficulties
Low socioeconomic class
Maladaptive coping strategies
Marital conflict
Mother of child not involved

Single parent
Social isolation
Poor home environment
Poor parental role model
Poor problem-solving skills
Poverty
Presence of stress (e.g., financial, legal, recent crisis, cultural move)
Relocations
Role strain
Situational low self-esteem
Unemployment
Unplanned pregnancy
Unwanted pregnancy

P

RISK FOR IMPAIRED PARENTING
(1978, 1998)

Definition *Risk for inability of the primary caretaker to create, maintain, or regain an environment that promotes the optimum growth and development of the child*

Risk Factors

Infant or Child

Altered perceptual abilities

Attention deficit hyperactivity disorder

Developmental delay

Difficult temperament

Handicapping condition

Illness

Multiple births

Not gender desired

Premature birth

Prolonged separation from parent

Temperamental conflicts with parental expectation

Knowledge

Deficient knowledge about child development

Deficient knowledge about child health maintenance

Deficient knowledge about parenting skills

Inability to respond to infant cues

Lack of cognitive readiness for parenthood

Low cognitive functioning

Low educational level or attainment

Poor communication skills

Preference for physical punishment

Unrealistic expectations of child

Physiological

Physical illness

Psychological

Closely spaced pregnancies

Depression

Difficult birthing process

Disability

High number of pregnancies

History of mental illness

History of substance abuse

Sleep deprivation

Sleep disruption

Young parental age

P

Social

Change in family unit
Chronic low self-esteem
Father of child not involved
Financial difficulties
History of being abused
History of being abusive
Inadequate child care arrangements
Job problems
Lack of access to resources
Lack of family cohesiveness
Lack of parental role model
Lack of prenatal care
Lack of resources
Lack of social support network
Lack of transportation
Lack of valuing of parenthood
Late prenatal care
Legal difficulties
Low socioeconomic class
Maladaptive coping strategies
Marital conflict
Mother of child not involved
Parent-child separation
Poor home environment
Poor parental role model
Poor problem-solving skills
Poverty
Role strain
Single parent
Situational low self-esteem
Social isolation
Stress
Relocation
Unemployment
Unplanned pregnancy
Unwanted pregnancy

P

RISK FOR PERIPHERAL NEUROVASCULAR DYSFUNCTION
(1992)

Definition *At risk for disruption in circulation, sensation, or motion of an extremity*

Risk Factors

Burns
Fractures
Immobilization
Mechanical compression
    (e.g., tourniquet, cane,
    cast, brace, dressing,
    restraint)
Orthopedic surgery
Trauma
Vascular obstruction

P

RISK FOR POISONING
(1980, 2006, LOE 2.1)

Definition *Accentuated risk of accidental exposure to, or ingestion of, drugs or dangerous products in doses sufficient to cause poisoning*

Risk Factors

External

Availability of illicit drugs potentially contaminated by poisonous additives

Dangerous products placed within reach of children

Dangerous products placed within reach of confused individuals

Large supplies of drugs in house

Medicines stored in unlocked cabinets accessible to children

Medicines stored in unlocked cabinets accessible to confused individuals

Internal

Cognitive difficulties

Emotional difficulties

Lack of drug education

Lack of proper precaution

Lack of safety education

Reduced vision

Verbalization that occupational setting is without adequate safeguards

Reference

Centers for Disease Control & Prevention. (2005). *Third national report on human exposure to environmental chemicals: Executive summary* (NCEH Pub # 05-0725). Atlanta: Author.

Post-trauma syndrome
(1986, 1998)

Definition *Sustained maladaptive response to a traumatic, overwhelming event*

Defining Characteristics

- Aggression
- Alienation
- Altered mood states
- Anger
- Anxiety
- Avoidance
- Compulsive behavior
- Denial
- Depression
- Detachment
- Difficulty concentrating
- Enuresis (in children)
- Exaggerated startle response
- Fear
- Flashbacks
- Gastric irritability
- Grieving
- Guilt
- Headaches
- Hopelessness
- Horror
- Hypervigilance
- Intrusive dreams
- Intrusive thoughts
- Irritability
- Neurosensory irritability
- Nightmares
- Palpitations
- Panic attacks
- Psychogenic amnesia
- Rage
- Rape
- Reports feeling numb
- Repression
- Shame
- Substance abuse

Related Factors

Abuse (physical and psychosocial)
Being held prisoner of war
Criminal victimization
Disasters
Epidemics
Events outside the range of usual human experience

Serious accidents (e.g., industrial, motor vehicle)
Serious injury to loved ones
Serious injury to self
Serious threat to loved ones
Serious threat to self

Sudden destruction of
  one's community
Sudden destruction of
  one's home
Torture
Tragic occurrence involv-
  ing multiple deaths
Wars
Witnessing mutilation
Witnessing violent death

P

RISK FOR POST-TRAUMA SYNDROME
(1998)

Definition *At risk for sustained maladaptive response to a traumatic, overwhelming event*

Risk Factors

Diminished ego strength
Displacement from home
Duration of the event
Exaggerated sense of responsibility
Inadequate social support
Nonsupportive environment

Occupation (e.g., police, fire, rescue, corrections, emergency room staff, mental health worker)
Perception of event
Survivor's role in the event

P

READINESS FOR ENHANCED POWER
(2006, LOE 2.1)

Definition   *A pattern of participating knowingly in change that is sufficient for well-being and can be strengthened*

Defining Characteristics

- Expresses readiness to enhance awareness of possible changes to be made
- Expresses readiness to enhance freedom to perform actions for change
- Expresses readiness to enhance identification of choices that can be made for change
- Expresses readiness to enhance involvement in creating change

- Expresses readiness to enhance knowledge for participation in change
- Expresses readiness to enhance participation in choices for daily living & health
- Expresses readiness to enhance power

References

Jeng, C., Yang, S., Chang, P., & Tsao, L. (2004). Menopausal women: Perceiving continuous power through the experience of regular exercise. *Journal of Clinical Nursing, 13,* 447-454.

Shearer, N., & Reed, P. (2004). Empowerment: Reformulation of a non-Rogerian concept. *Nursing Science Quarterly, 17,* 253-259.

Wright, B. (2004). Trust and power in adults: An investigation using Rogers' science of unitary human beings. *Nursing Science Quarterly, 17,* 139-146.

P

Note. Even though power (a response) and empowerment (an intervention approach) are different concepts, the literature related to both concepts supports the defining characteristics of this diagnosis.

POWERLESSNESS
(1982)

Definition   *Perception that one's own action will not significantly affect an outcome; a perceived lack of control over a current situation or immediate happening*

Defining Characteristics

Low
- Expressions of uncertainty about fluctuating energy levels
- Passivity

Moderate
- Anger
- Dependence on others that may result in irritability
- Does not defend self-care practices when challenged
- Does not monitor progress
- Expressions of dissatisfaction over inability to perform previous tasks/activities
- Expressions of doubt regarding role performance
- Expressions of frustration over inability to perform previous tasks/activities
- Fear of alienation from caregivers

- Guilt
- Inability to seek information regarding care
- Nonparticipation in care when opportunities are provided
- Nonparticipation in decision making when opportunities are provided
- Passivity
- Reluctance to express true feelings
- Resentment

Severe
- Apathy
- Depression over physical deterioration
- Verbal expressions of having no control (e.g., over self-care, situation, outcome)

Related Factors

Healthcare environment
Illness-related regimen

Interpersonal interaction
Lifestyle of helplessness

RISK FOR POWERLESSNESS
(2000)

Definition   *At risk for perceived lack of control over a situation and/or one's ability to significantly affect an outcome*

Risk Factors

Physiological

Acute injury
Aging
Dying
Illness
Progressive debilitating disease process (e.g., spinal cord injury, multiple sclerosis)

Psychosocial

Absence of integrality (e.g., essence of power)

Chronic low self-esteem
Deficient knowledge (e.g., of illness or healthcare system)
Disturbed body image
Inadequate coping patterns
Lifestyle of dependency
Situational low self-esteem

P

INEFFECTIVE PROTECTION
(1990)

Definition *Decrease in the ability to guard self from internal or external threats such as illness or injury*

Defining Characteristics
- Altered clotting
- Anorexia
- Chilling
- Cough
- Deficient immunity
- Disorientation
- Dyspnea
- Fatigue
- Immobility
- Impaired healing
- Insomnia
- Itching
- Maladaptive stress response
- Neurosensory alteration
- Perspiring
- Pressure ulcers
- Restlessness
- Weakness

Related Factors
Abnormal blood profiles (e.g., leukopenia, thrombocytopenia, anemia, coagulation)
Alcohol abuse
Cancer
Drug therapies (e.g., antineoplastic, corticosteroid, immune, anticoagulant, thrombolytic)

Extremes of age
Immune disorders
Inadequate nutrition
Treatments (e.g., surgery, radiation)

Rape-Trauma Syndrome
(1980, 1998)

Definition *Sustained maladaptive response to a forced, violent sexual penetration against the victim's will and consent*

Defining Characteristics

- Aggression
- Agitation
- Anger
- Anxiety
- Change in relationships
- Confusion
- Denial
- Dependence
- Depression
- Disorganization
- Dissociative disorders
- Embarrassment
- Fear
- Guilt
- Helplessness
- Humiliation
- Hyperalertness
- Impaired decision making
- Loss of self-esteem
- Mood swings
- Muscle spasms
- Muscle tension
- Nightmares
- Paranoia
- Phobias
- Physical trauma
- Powerlessness
- Revenge
- Self-blame
- Sexual dysfunction
- Shame
- Shock
- Sleep disturbances
- Substance abuse
- Suicide attempts
- Vulnerability

Related Factors

Rape

Note. This syndrome includes the following three subcomponents: Rape-Trauma, Compound Reaction, and Silent Reaction. In this text each appears as a separate diagnosis.

Rape-Trauma Syndrome: Compound Reaction
(1980)

Definition *Forced violent sexual penetration against the victim's will and consent. The trauma syndrome that develops from this attack or attempted attack includes an acute phase of disorganization of the victim's lifestyle and a long-term process of reorganization of lifestyle.*

Defining Characteristics

- Change in lifestyle (e.g., changes in residence, dealing with repetitive nightmares and phobias, seeking family support, seeking social network support in long-term phase)
- Emotional reaction (e.g., anger, embarrassment, fear of physical violence and death, humiliation, revenge, self-blame in acute phase)
- Multiple physical symptoms (e.g., gastrointestinal irritability, genitourinary discomfort, muscle tension, sleep pattern disturbance in acute phase)
- Reactivated symptoms of previous conditions (e.g., physical illness, psychiatric illness in acute phase)
- Substance abuse (acute phase)

Related Factors
To be developed

Note. This syndrome includes the following three subcomponents: Rape-Trauma, Compound Reaction, and Silent Reaction. In this text each appears as a separate diagnosis. This diagnosis will retire from the NANDA-I Taxonomy in the 2009–2010 edition unless additional work is done to bring it to a LOE of 2.1 or higher.

Rape-trauma syndrome: silent reaction
(1980)

Definition   *Forced violent sexual penetration against the victim's will and consent. The trauma syndrome that develops from this attack or attempted attack includes an acute phase of disorganization of the victim's lifestyle and a long-term process of reorganization of lifestyle.*

Defining Characteristics

- Abrupt changes in relationships with men
- Increase in nightmares
- Increased anxiety during interview (e.g., blocking of associations, long periods of silence, minor stuttering, physical distress)
- No verbalization of the occurrence of rape
- Pronounced changes in sexual behavior
- Sudden onset of phobic reactions

Related Factors

To be developed

R

Note. This syndrome includes the following three subcomponents: Rape-Trauma, Compound Reaction, and Silent Reaction. In this text each appears as a separate diagnosis. This diagnosis will retire from the NANDA-I Taxonomy in the 2009–2010 edition unless additional work is done to bring it to a LOE of 2.1 or higher.

IMPAIRED RELIGIOSITY*
(2004, LOE 2.1)

Definition *Impaired ability to exercise reliance on beliefs and/or participate in rituals of a particular faith tradition*

Defining Characteristics

- Difficulty adhering to prescribed religions beliefs and rituals (e.g., religious ceremonies, dietary regulations, clothing, prayer, worship/religious services, private religious behaviors/reading religious materials/media, holiday observances, meetings with religious leaders)
- Expresses emotional distress because of separation from faith community
- Expresses a need to reconnect with previous belief patterns
- Expresses a need to reconnect with previous customs
- Questions religious belief patterns
- Questions religious customs

Related Factors

Developmental & Situational

Aging
End-stage life crises
Life transitions

Physical

Illness
Pain

---

* *The DDC recognizes that the term "religiosity" may be culture specific; however, the term is useful in the U.S. and is well-supported in the U.S. literature.*

Psychological

Anxiety
Fear of death
Ineffective coping
Ineffective support
Lack of security
Personal crisis
Use of religion to manip-
ulate

Sociocultural

Cultural barriers to practicing religion
Environmental barriers
to practicing religion
Lack of social integration
Lack of sociocultural
interaction

Spiritual

Spiritual crises
Suffering

R

READINESS FOR ENHANCED RELIGIOSITY*
(2004, LOE 2.1)

Definition *Ability to increase reliance on religious beliefs and/or participate in rituals of a particular faith tradition*

Defining Characteristics

- Expresses desire to strengthen religious belief patterns that had provided comfort in the past
- Expresses desire to strengthen religious belief patterns that had provided religion in the past
- Expresses desire to strengthen religious customs that had provided comfort in the past
- Expresses desire to strengthen religious customs that had provided religion in the past
- Questions belief patterns that are harmful
- Questions customs that are harmful
- Rejects belief patterns that are harmful
- Rejects customs that are harmful

- Requests assistance expanding religious options
- Request for assistance to increase participation in prescribed religious beliefs (e.g., religious ceremonies, dietary regulations/rituals, clothing, prayer, worship/religious services, private religious behaviors, reading religious materials/media, holiday observances)
- Requests forgiveness
- Requests meeting with religious leaders/facilitators
- Requests reconciliation
- Requests religious experiences
- Requests religious materials

* *The DDC recognizes that the term "religiosity" may be culture specific; however, the term is useful in the U.S. and is well-supported in the U.S. literature.*

RISK FOR IMPAIRED Rᴇʟɪɢɪᴏsɪᴛʏ*
(2004, ʟᴏᴇ 2.1)

Definition *At risk for an impaired ability to exercise reliance on religious beliefs and/or participate in rituals of a particular faith tradition*

Related Factors

Developmental

Life transitions

Environmental

Barriers to practicing religion

Lack of transportation

Physical

Hospitalization
Illness
Pain

Psychological

Depression
Ineffective caregiving
Ineffective coping
Ineffective support
Lack of security

Sociocultural

Cultural barrier to practicing religion
Lack of social interaction
Social isolation

Spiritual

Suffering

R

---

* *The DDC recognizes that the term "religiosity" may be culture specific; however, the term is useful in the U.S. and is well-supported in the U.S. literature.*

RELOCATION STRESS SYNDROME
(1992, 2000)

Definition *Physiological and/or psychosocial disturbance following transfer from one environment to another*

Defining Characteristics

- Alienation
- Aloneness
- Anger
- Anxiety (e.g., separation)
- Concern over relocation
- Dependency
- Depression
- Fear
- Frustration
- Increased illness
- Increased physical symptoms
- Increased verbalization of needs
- Insecurity
- Loneliness
- Loss of identity
- Loss of self-esteem
- Loss of self-worth
- Move from one environment to another
- Pessimism
- Sleep disturbance
- Unwillingness to move
- Withdrawal
- Worry

Related Factors

Decreased health status
Feelings of powerlessness
Unpredictability of experience
Impaired psychosocial health
Isolation
Lack of adequate support system
Lack of predeparture counseling
Language barrier
Losses
Passive coping

R

RISK FOR RELOCATION STRESS SYNDROME
(2000)

Definition   *At risk for physiological and/or psychosocial disturbance following transfer from one environment to another*

Risk Factors

Decreased health status
Feelings of powerlessness
Lack of adequate support
  system
Lack of predeparture
  counseling
Losses
Moderate to high degree
  of environmental
  change
Moderate mental competence
Move from one environment to another
Passive coping
Unpredictability of experiences

INEFFECTIVE ROLE PERFORMANCE
(1978, 1996, 1998)

Definition *Patterns of behavior and self-expression that do not match the environmental context, norms, and expectations*

Defining Characteristics

- Altered role perceptions
- Anxiety
- Change in capacity to resume role
- Change in other's perception of role
- Change in self-perception of role
- Change in usual patterns of responsibility
- Deficient knowledge
- Depression
- Discrimination
- Domestic violence
- Harassment
- Inadequate adaptation to change
- Inadequate confidence
- Inadequate coping
- Inappropriate developmental expectations
- Inadequate external support for role enactment
- Inadequate motivation
- Inadequate opportunities for role enactment
- Inadequate role competency
- Inadequate self-management
- Inadequate skills
- Pessimism
- Powerlessness
- Role ambivalence
- Role confusion
- Role conflict
- Role denial
- Role dissatisfaction
- Role overload
- Role strain
- System conflict
- Uncertainty

Related Factors

Knowledge

Inadequate role model
Inadequate role preparation (e.g., role transition, skill rehearsal, validation)

Lack of education
Lack of role model
Unrealistic role expectations

Physiological

Body image alteration
Cognitive deficits
Depression
Fatigue
Low self-esteem
Mental illness
Neurological defects
Pain
Physical illness
Substance abuse

Social

Conflict
Developmental level
Domestic violence
Inadequate role socialization
Inadequate support system
Inappropriate linkage with the healthcare system
Job schedule demands
Lack of resources
Lack of rewards
Low socioeconomic status
Stress
Young age

R

S

READINESS FOR ENHANCED SELF-CARE
(2006, LOE 2.1)

Definition *A pattern of performing activities for oneself that helps to meet health-related goals and can be strengthened*

Defining Characteristics

- Expresses desire to enhance independence in maintaining life
- Expresses desire to enhance independence in maintaining health
- Expresses desire to enhance independence in maintaining personal development
- Expresses desire to enhance independence in maintaining well-being
- Expresses desire to enhance knowledge of strategies for self-care
- Expresses desire to enhance responsibility for self-care
- Expresses desire to enhance self-care

References

Becker, G., Gates, R. J., & Newsom, E. (2004). Self-care among chronically ill African Americans: Culture, health disparities, and health insurance status. *American Journal of Public Health, 94*, 2066-2073.

Dashiff, C., Bartolucci, A., Wallander, J., & Abdullatif, H. (2005). The relationship of family structure, maternal employment, and family conflict with self-care adherence of adolescents with type 1 diabetes. *Families, Systems, & Health, 23*(1), 66-79.

Orem, D.E. (2001). *Nursing: Concepts and practice* (6th ed.) St. Louis: Mosby.

BATHING/HYGIENE Sᴇʟꜰ-CARE DEFICIT
(1980, 1998)

Definition *Impaired ability to perform or complete bathing/hygiene activities for oneself*

Defining Characteristics
- Inability to access bathroom
- Inability to dry body
- Inability to get bath supplies
- Inability to obtain water source
- Inability to regulate bath water
- Inability to wash body

Related Factors
Cognitive impairment
Decreased motivation
Environmental barriers
Inability to perceive body part
Inability to perceive spatial relationship
Musculoskeletal impairment
Neuromuscular impairment
Pain
Perceptual impairment
Severe anxiety
Weakness

S

Note. Specify level of independence using a standardized functional scale.

DRESSING/GROOMING Self-CARE DEFICIT
(1980, 1998)

Definition *Impaired ability to perform or complete dressing and grooming activities for self*

Defining Characteristics

- Inability to choose clothing
- Inability to put clothing on lower body
- Inability to maintain appearance at a satisfactory level
- Inability to pick up clothing
- Inability to put clothing on upper body
- Inability to put on shoes
- Inability to put on socks
- Inability to remove clothes
- Inability to use assistive devices
- Inability to use zippers
- Impaired ability to fasten clothing
- Impaired ability to obtain clothing
- Impaired ability to put on necessary items of clothing
- Impaired ability to take off necessary items of clothing

Related Factors

Cognitive impairment
Decreased motivation
Discomfort
Environmental barriers
Fatique
Musculoskeletal impairment

Neuromuscular impairment
Pain
Perceptual impairment
Severe anxiety
Weakness

Note. Specify level of independence using a standardized functional scale.

FEEDING SELF-CARE DEFICIT
(1980, 1998)

Definition *Impaired ability to perform or complete feeding activities*

Defining Characteristics

- Inability to bring food from a receptacle to the mouth
- Inability to chew food
- Inability to complete a meal
- Inability to get food onto utensil
- Inability to handle utensils
- Inability to ingest food in a socially acceptable manner
- Inability to ingest food safely
- Inability to ingest sufficient food
- Inability to manipulate food in mouth
- Inability to open containers
- Inability to pick up cup or glass
- Inability to prepare food for ingestion
- Inability to swallow food
- Inability to use assistive device

Related Factors

Cognitive impairment
Decreased motivation
Discomfort
Environmental barriers
Fatigue
Musculoskeletal impairment
Neuromuscular impairment
Pain
Perceptual impairment
Severe anxiety
Weakness

S

Note. Specify level of independence using a standardized functional scale.

TOILETING SELF-CARE DEFICIT
(1980, 1998)

Definition *Impaired ability to perform or complete own toileting activities*

Defining Characteristics

- Inability to carry out proper toilet hygiene
- Inability to flush toilet or commode
- Inability to get to toilet or commode
- Inability to manipulate clothing for toileting
- Inability to rise from toilet or commode
- Inability to sit on toilet or commode

Related Factors

Cognitive impairment
Decreased motivation
Environmental barriers
Fatique
Impaired mobility status
Impaired transfer ability
Musculoskeletal impairment

Neuromuscular impairment
Pain
Perceptual impairment
Severe anxiety
Weakness

S

Note. Specify level of independence using a standardized functional scale.

READINESS FOR ENHANCED SELF-CONCEPT

(2002, LOE 2.1)

Definition *A pattern of perceptions or ideas about the self that is sufficient for well-being and can be strengthened*

Defining Characteristics

- Accepts limitations
- Accepts strengths
- Actions are congruent with verbal expression
- Expresses confidence in abilities
- Expresses satisfaction with body image
- Expresses satisfaction with personal identity
- Expresses satisfaction with role performance
- Expresses satisfaction with sense of worthiness
- Expresses satisfaction with thoughts about self
- Expresses willingness to enhance self-concept

S

CHRONIC LOW SELF-ESTEEM
(1988, 1996)

Definition *Long-standing negative self-evaluation/feelings about self or self-capabilities*

Defining Characteristics

- Dependent on others' opinions
- Evaluates self as unable to deal with events
- Exaggerates negative feedback about self
- Excessively seeks reassurance
- Expressions of guilt
- Expressions of shame
- Frequent lack of success in life events
- Hesitant to try new things/situations
- Indecisive
- Lack of eye contact
- Nonassertive
- Overly conforming
- Passive
- Rejects positive feedback about self
- Self-negating verbalization

Related Factors

To be developed

S

Note. *This diagnosis will retire from the NANDA-I Taxonomy in the 2009–2010 edition unless additional work is done to bring it to a LOE of 2.1 or higher.*

SITUATIONAL LOW SELF-ESTEEM
(1988, 1996, 2000)

Definition *Development of a negative perception of self-worth in response to a current situation (specify)*

Defining Characteristics

- Evaluation of self as unable to deal with situations or events
- Expressions of helplessness
- Expressions of uselessness
- Indecisive behavior
- Nonassertive behavior
- Self-negating verbalizations
- Verbally reports current situational challenge to self-worth

Related Factors

Behavior inconsistent with values
Developmental changes
Disturbed body image
Failures

Functional impairment
Lack of recognition
Loss
Rejections
Social role changes

S

RISK FOR SITUATIONAL LOW SELF-ESTEEM
(2000)

Definition *At risk for developing negative perception of self-worth in response to a current situation (specify)*

Risk Factors

Behavior inconsistent
with values
Decreased control over
environment
Developmental changes
Disturbed body image
Failures
Functional impairment
History of abandonment
History of abuse
History of learned help-
lessness

History of neglect
Lack of recognition
Loss
Physical illness
Rejections
Social role changes
Unrealistic self-expecta-
tions

S

SELF-MUTILATION
(2000)

Definition   *Deliberate self-injurious behavior causing tissue damage with the intent of causing nonfatal injury to attain relief of tension*

Defining Characteristics

- Abrading
- Biting
- Constricting a body part
- Cuts on body
- Hitting
- Ingestion of harmful substances
- Inhalation of harmful substances
- Insertion of object into body orifice
- Picking at wounds
- Scratches on body
- Self-inflicted burns
- Severing

Related Factors

Adolescence
Autistic individual
Battered child
Borderline personality disorder
Character disorder
Childhood illness
Childhood sexual abuse
Childhood surgery
Depersonalization
Developmentally delayed individual
Dissociation
Disturbed body image
Disturbed interpersonal relationships
Eating disorders
Emotionally disturbed

Family alcoholism
Family divorce
Family history of self-destructive behaviors
Feels threatened with loss of significant relationship
History of inability to plan solutions
History of inability to see long-term consequences
History of self-injurious behavior
Impulsivity
Inability to express tension verbally
Incarceration

continued

Self-Mutilation,   *continued*

Ineffective coping
Irresistible urge to cut/
   damage self
Isolation from peers
Labile behavior
Lack of family confidant
Living in nontraditional
   setting (e.g., foster,
   group, or institutional
   care)
Low self-esteem
Mounting tension that is
   intolerable
Needs quick reduction of
   stress
Negative feelings (e.g.,
   depression, rejection,
   self-hatred, separation
   anxiety, guilt, deper-
   sonalization)

Peers who self-mutilate
Perfectionism
Poor communication
   between parent and
   adolescent
Psychotic state (e.g., com-
   mand hallucinations)
Sexual identity crisis
Substance abuse
Unstable body image
Unstable self-esteem
Use of manipulation to
   obtain nurturing rela-
   tionship with others
Violence between
   parental figures

S

RISK FOR SELF-MUTILATION
(1992, 2000)

Definition   *At risk for deliberate self-injurious behavior caus-ing tissue damage with the intent of causing nonfatal injury to attain relief of tension*

Risk Factors

Adolescence

Autistic individuals

Battered child

Borderline personality disorders

Character disorders

Childhood illness

Childhood sexual abuse

Childhood surgery

Depersonalization

Developmentally delayed individuals

Dissociation

Disturbed body image

Disturbed interpersonal relationships

Eating disorders

Emotionally disturbed child

Family alcoholism

Family divorce

Family history of self-destructive behaviors

Feels threatened with loss of significant relationship

History of inability to plan solutions

History of inability to see long-term consequences

History of self-injurious behavior

Impulsivity

Inability to express tension verbally

Inadequate coping

Incarceration

Irresistible urge to damage self

Isolation from peers

Living in nontraditional setting (e.g., foster, group, or institutional care)

Loss of control over problem-solving situations

Low self-esteem

Loss of significant relationship(s)

Mounting tension that is intolerable

Needs quick reduction of stress

continued

Risk for Self-Mutilation, *continued*

Negative feelings (e.g., depression, rejection, self-hatred, separation anxiety, guilt)

Peers who self-mutilate

Perfectionism

Psychotic state (e.g., command hallucinations)

Sexual identity crisis

Substance abuse

Unstable self-esteem

Use of manipulation to obtain nurturing relationship with others

Violence between parental figures

S

DISTURBED Sensory PERCEPTION
(Specify: Visual, Auditory, Kinesthetic, Gustatory, Tactile, Olfactory)
(1978, 1980, 1998)

Definition *Change in the amount or patterning of incoming stimuli accompanied by a diminished, exaggerated, distorted, or impaired response to such stimuli*

Defining Characteristics

- Change in behavior pattern
- Change in problem-solving abilities
- Change in sensory acuity
- Change in usual response to stimuli
- Disorientation

- Hallucinations
- Impaired communication
- Irritability
- Poor concentration
- Restlessness
- Sensory distortions

Related Factors

Altered sensory integration
Altered sensory reception
Altered sensory transmission
Biochemical imbalance

Electrolyte imbalance
Excessive environmental stimuli
Insufficient environmental stimuli
Psychological stress

S

Sexual dysfunction
(1980, 2006, LOE 2.1)

Definition *The state in which an individual experiences a change in sexual function during the sexual response phases of desire, excitation, and/or orgasm, which is viewed as unsatisfying, unrewarding or inadequate*

Defining Characteristics

- Alterations in achieving sexual satisfaction
- Alterations in achieving perceived sex role
- Actual limitations imposed by disease
- Actual limitations imposed by therapy
- Change of interest in others
- Change of interest in self
- Inability to achieve desired satisfaction
- Perceived alteration in sexual excitation
- Perceived deficiency of sexual desire
- Perceived limitations imposed by disease
- Perceived limitations imposed by therapy
- Seeking confirmation of desirability
- Verbalization of problem

Related Factors

Absent role models
Altered body function (e.g. pregnancy, recent childbirth, drugs, surgery, anomalies, disease process, trauma, radiation)
Altered body structure (e.g. pregnancy, recent childbirth, surgery, anomalies, disease process, trauma, radiation)

Biopsychosocial alteration of sexuality
Ineffectual role models
Lack of privacy
Lack of significant other
Misinformation or lack of knowledge
Values conflict
Psychosocial abuse (e.g., harmful relationships)
Physical abuse
Vulnerability

References

Hogan, R.M. (1985). *Human sexuality–A nursing perspective.* New York: Appleton-Century-Crofts.

Kolodny, R C., Masters, W.H., & Johnson, V.E. (1979). *Textbook of sexual medicine.* Boston: Little, Brown.

Kaplan, H.S. *(1983). O desejo sexual ñ e novos conceitos etÈcnicas da terapia do sexo.* Rio de Janeiro: Nova Fronteira.

S

INEFFECTIVE SEXUALITY PATTERN
(1986, 2006, LOE 2.1)

Definition *Expressions of concern regarding own sexuality*

Defining Characteristics

- Alterations in achieving perceived sex role
- Alteration in relationship with significant other
- Conflicts involving values
- Reported changes in sexual activities
- Reported changes in sexual behaviors
- Reported difficulties in sexual behaviors
- Reported difficulties in sexual activities
- Reported limitations in sexual behaviors
- Reported limitations in sexual activities

Related Factors

Absent role model

Conflicts with sexual orientation or variant preferences

Fear of acquiring a sexually transmitted disease

Fear of pregnancy

Impaired relationship with a significant other

Ineffective role model

Knowledge/skill deficit about alternative responses to health-related transitions, altered body function or structure, illness, or medical treatment

Lack of privacy

Lack of significant other

S

References

Hogan, R.M. (1985). *Human sexuality–A nursing perspective.* New York: Appleton-Century-Crofts.

Kolodny, R C., Masters, W.H., & Johnson, V.E. (1979). *Textbook of sexual medicine.* Boston: Little, Brown.

Kaplan, H.S. *n(1983). O desejo sexual – e novos conceitos etécnicas da terapia do sexo.* Rio de Janeiro: Nova Fronteira.

IMPAIRED SKIN INTEGRITY
(1975, 1998)

Definition   *Altered epidermis and/or dermis*

Defining Characteristics
- Destruction of skin layers
- Disruption of skin surface
- Invasion of body structures

Related Factors

External

Chemical substance
Extremes in age
Humidity
Hyperthermia
Hypothermia
Mechanical factors (e.g., shearing forces, pressure, restraint)
Medications
Moisture
Physical immobilization
Radiation

Internal

Changes in fluid status
Changes in pigmentation
Changes in turgor
Developmental factors
Imbalanced nutritional state (e.g., obesity, emaciation)
Immunological deficit
Impaired circulation
Impaired metabolic state
Impaired sensation
Skeletal prominence

S

RISK FOR IMPAIRED SKIN INTEGRITY
(1975, 1998)

Definition   *At risk for skin being adversely altered*

Risk Factors

External

Chemical substance
Excretions
Extremes of age
Hyperthermia
Hypothermia
Humidity
Mechanical factors (e.g., shearing forces, pressure, restraint)
Moisture
Physical immobilization
Radiation
Secretions

Internal

Changes in pigmentation
Changes in skin turgor
Developmental factors
Imbalanced nutritional state (e.g., obesity, emaciation)
Impaired circulation
Impaired metabolic state
Impaired sensation
Immunologic factors
Medications
Psychogenetic factors
Skeletal prominence

S

Note. Risk should be determined by use of a standardized risk assessment tool.

SLEEP DEPRIVATION
(1998)

Definition   *Prolonged periods of time without sleep (sustained natural, periodic suspension of relative consciousness)*

Defining Characteristics

- Acute confusion
- Agitation
- Anxiety
- Apathy
- Combativeness
- Daytime drowsiness
- Decreased ability to function
- Fatique
- Fleeting nystagmus
- Hallucinations
- Hand tremors
- Heightened sensitivity to pain
- Inability to concentrate
- Irritability
- Lethargy
- Listlessness
- Malaise
- Perceptual disorders (e.g., disturbed body sensation, delusions, feeling afloat)
- Restlessness
- Slowed reaction
- Transient paranoia

Related Factors

Aging-related sleep stage shifts
Dementia
Familial sleep paralysis
Inadequate daytime activity
Idiopathic central nervous system hypersomnolence
Narcolepsy
Nightmares
Non-sleep-inducing parenting practices
Periodic limb movement (e.g., restless leg syndrome, nocturnal myoclonus)
Prolonged discomfort (e.g., physical, psychological)
Sustained inadequate sleep hygiene
Prolonged use of pharmacologic or dietary antisoporifics
Sleep apnea

continued

Sleep Deprivation, *continued*

Sleep terror
Sleep walking
Sleep-related enuresis
Sleep-related painful
  erections
Sundowner's syndrome
Sustained circadian asyn-
  chrony
Sustained environmental
  stimulation
Sustained uncomfortable
  sleep environment

S

READINESS FOR ENHANCED SLEEP
(2002, LOE 2.1)

Definition *A pattern of natural, periodic suspension of consciousness that provides adequate rest, sustains a desired lifestyle, and can be strengthened*

Defining Characteristics

- Amount of sleep is congruent with developmental needs
- Expresses a feeling of being rested after sleep
- Expresses willingness to enhance sleep
- Follows sleep routines that promote sleep habits
- Occasional use of medications to induce sleep

S

IMPAIRED SOCIAL INTERACTION
(1986)

Definition *Insufficient or excessive quantity or ineffective quality of social exchange*

Defining Characteristics

- Discomfort in social situations
- Dysfunctional interaction with others
- Family report of changes in interaction (e.g., style, pattern)
- Inability to communicate a satisfying sense of social engagement (e.g., belonging, caring, interest, or shared history)
- Inability to receive a satisfying sense of social engagement (e.g., belonging, caring, interest, or shared history)
- Use of unsuccessful social interaction behaviors

Related Factors

Absence of significant others
Communication barriers
Deficit about ways to enhance mutuality (e.g., knowledge, skills)
Disturbed thought processes

Environmental barriers
Limited physical mobility
Self-concept disturbance
Sociocultural dissonance
Therapeutic isolation

S

SOCIAL ISOLATION
(1982)

Definition   *Aloneness experienced by the individual and perceived as imposed by others and as a negative or threatening state*

Defining Characteristics

Objective

- Absence of supportive significant other (s)
- Developmentally inappropriate behaviors
- Dull affect
- Evidence of handicap (e.g., physical, mental)
- Exists in a subculture
- Illness
- Meaningless actions
- No eye contact
- Preoccupation with own thoughts
- Projects hostility
- Repetitive actions
- Sad affect
- Seeks to be alone
- Shows behavior unaccepted by dominant cultural group
- Uncommunicative
- Withdrawn

Subjective

- Expresses feelings of aloneness imposed by others
- Expresses feelings of rejection
- Developmentally inappropriate interests
- Inadequate purpose in life
- Inability to meet expectations of others
- Expresses values unacceptable to the dominant cultural group
- Experiences feelings of differences from others
- Insecurity in public

continued

S

Social Isolation, *continued*

Related Factors

Alterations in mental status

Alterations in physical appearance

Altered state of wellness

Factors contributing to the absence of satisfying personal relationships (e.g., delay in accomplishing developmental tasks)

Immature interests

Inability to engage in satisfying personal relationships

Inadequate personal resources

Unaccepted social values

Unaccepted social behavior

S

CHRONIC SORROW
(1998)

Definition *Cyclical, recurring, and potentially progressive pattern of pervasive sadness experienced (by a parent, caregiver, individual with chronic illness or disability) in response to continual loss, throughout the trajectory of an illness or disability*

Defining Characteristics

- Expresses negative feelings (e.g., anger, being misunderstood, confusion, depression, disappointment, emptiness, fear, frustration, guilt, self-blame, helplessness, hopelessness, loneliness, low self-esteem, recurring loss, overwhelmed)
- Expresses feelings of sadness (e.g., periodic, recurrent)
- Expresses feelings that interfere with ability to reach highest level of personal well-being
- Expresses feelings that interfere with ability to reach highest level of social well-being

Related Factors

Death of a loved one
Experiences chronic disability (e.g., physical or mental)
Experiences chronic illness (e.g., physical or mental)
Crises in management of the illness
Crises related to developmental stages
Missed opportunities
Missed milestones
Unending caregiving

S

SPIRITUAL DISTRESS
(1978, 2002, LOE 2.1)

Definition *Impaired ability to experience and integrate meaning and purpose in life through connectedness with self, others, art, music, literature, nature, and/or a power greater than oneself*

Defining Characteristics

Connections to Self

- Anger
- Expresses lack of acceptance
- Expresses lack of courage
- Expresses lack of forgiveness of self
- Expresses lack of hope
- Expresses lack of love
- Expresses lack of meaning in life
- Expresses lack of purpose in life
- Expresses lack of serenity (e.g., peace)
- Guilt
- Poor coping

Connections With Others

- Expresses alienation
- Refuses interactions with significant others
- Refuses interactions with spiritual leaders
- Verbalizes being separated from support system

Connections With Art, Music, Literature, Nature

- Disinterest in nature
- Disinterest in reading spiritual literature
- Inability to express previous state of creativity (e.g., singing/listening to music/writing)

Connections With Power Greater Than Self

- Expresses being abandoned
- Expresses having anger toward God
- Expresses hopelessness
- Expresses suffering
- Inability to be introspective
- Inability to experience the transcendent
- Inability to participate in religious activities
- Inability to pray

- Requests to see a religious leader
- Sudden changes in spiritual practices

Related Factors

Active dying
Anxiety
Chronic illness
Death
Life change

Loneliness
Pain
Self-alienation
Social alienation
Sociocultural deprivation

S

RISK FOR SPIRITUAL DISTRESS
(1998, 2004, LOE 2.1)

Definition *At risk for an impaired ability to experience and integrate meaning and purpose in life through connectedness with self, others, art, music, literature, nature, and/or a power greater than oneself*

Risk Factors

Developmental

Life changes

Environmental

Environmental changes
Natural disasters

Physical

Chronic illness
Physical illness
Substance abuse

Psychosocial

Anxiety
Blocks to experiencing love

Change in religious rituals
Change in spiritual practices
Cultural conflict
Depression
Inability to forgive
Loss
Low self-esteem
Poor relationships
Racial conflict
Separated support systems
Stress

S

READINESS FOR ENHANCED Spiritual WELL-BEING
(1994, 2002, loe 2.1)

Definition *Ability to experience and integrate meaning and purpose in life through connectedness with self, others, art, music, literature, nature, and/or a power greater than oneself that can be strengthened*

Defining Characteristics

Connections to Self

- Expresses desire for enhanced acceptance
- Expresses desire for enhanced coping
- Expresses desire for enhanced courage
- Expresses desire for enhanced forgiveness of self
- Expresses desire for enhanced hope
- Expresses desire for enhanced joy
- Expresses desire for enhanced love
- Expresses desire for enhanced meaning in life
- Expresses desire for enhanced purpose in life
- Expresses desire for enhanced satisfying philosophy of life
- Expresses desire for enhanced surrender
- Expresses lack of serenity (e.g., peace)
- Meditation

Connections With Others

- Provides service to others
- Requests interactions with significant others
- Requests interactions with spiritual leaders
- Requests forgiveness of others

Connections With Art, Music, Literature, Nature

- Displays creative energy (e.g., writing, poetry, singing)
- Listens to music
- Reads spiritual literature
- Spends time outdoors

Connections With Power Greater Than Self

- Expresses awe
- Expresses reverence
- Participates in religious activities
- Prays
- Reports mystical experiences

S

Sᴛʀᴇss OVERLOAD
(2006, ʟᴏᴇ 3.2)

Definition *Excessive amounts and types of demands that require action*

Defining Characteristics

- Demonstrates increased feelings of anger
- Demonstrates increased feelings of impatience
- Expresses difficulty in functioning
- Expresses a feeling of pressure
- Expresses a feeling of tension
- Expresses increased feelings of anger
- Expresses increased feelings of impatience
- Expresses problems with decision making
- Reports negative impact from stress (e.g., physical symptoms, psychological distress, feeling of "being sick" or of "going to get sick")
- Reports situational stress as excessive (e.g., rates stress level as seven or above on a 10-point scale)

Related Factors

Inadequate resources (e.g., financial, social, education/knowledge level)
Intense, repeated stressors (e.g., family violence, chronic illness, terminal illness)

Multiple coexisting stressors (e.g., environmental threats/demands; physical threats/demands; (social threats/demands)

S

References

Keil, R.M.K. (2004). Coping and stress: A conceptual analysis. *Journal of Advanced Nursing, 45*, 659-665.

Motzer, S.A., & Hertig, V. (2004). Stress, stress response and health. Nursing *Clinics of North America, 39*, 1-17.

Ryan-Wenger, N.A., Sharrer, V.W., & Campbell, K.K. (2005). Changes in children's stressors over the past 30 years. *Pediatric Nursing, 31*, 282-291.

S

RISK FOR SUFFOCATION
(1980)

Definition *Accentuated risk of accidental suffocation (inadequate air available for inhalation)*

Risk Factors

External

Discarding refrigerators
 without removed doors
Eating large mouthfuls of
 food
Hanging a pacifier
 around infant's neck
Household gas leaks
Inserting small objects
 into airway
Leaving children unat-
 tended in water
Low-strung clothesline
Pillow placed in infant's
 crib
Playing with plastic bags
Propped bottle placed in
 infant's crib
Smoking in bed
Use of fuel-burning
 heaters not vented to
 outside
Vehicle warming in
 closed garage

Internal

Cognitive difficulties
Disease process
Emotional difficulties
Injury process
Lack of safety education
Lack of safety precautions
Reduced motor abilities
Reduced olfactory
 sensation

S

RISK FOR SUICIDE
(2000)

Definition   *At risk for self-inflicted, life-threatening injury*

Risk Factors

Behavioral

Buying a gun
Changing a will
Giving away possessions
History of prior suicide
  attempt
Impulsiveness
Making a will
Marked changes in
  attitude
Marked changes in
  behavior
Marked changes in
  school performance
Stockpiling medicines
Sudden euphoric recovery
  from major depression

Demographic

Age (e.g., elderly, young
  adult males, adolescents)
Divorced
Male gender
Race (e.g., Caucasian,
Native American)
Widowed

Physical

Chronic pain
Physical illness
Terminal illness

Psychological

Childhood abuse
Family history of suicide
Gay or lesbian youth
Guilt
Psychiatric illness/disor-
  der (e.g., depression,
  schizophrenia, bipolar
  disorder)
Substance abuse

Situational

Adolescents living in
  nontraditional settings
  (e.g., juvenile detention
  center, prison, half-way
  house, group home)
Economic instability
Institutionalization
Living alone
Loss of autonomy
Loss of independence
Presence of gun in home
Relocation
Retired

continued

S

Risk for Suicide, *continued*

Social
Cluster suicides
Disrupted family life
Disciplinary problems
Grief
Helplessness
Hopelessness
Legal problems
Loneliness
Loss of important rela-
tionship
Poor support systems
Social isolation

Verbal
States desire to die
Threats of killing oneself

S

DELAYED SURGICAL RECOVERY
(1998, 2006, LOE 2.1)

Definition *Extension of the number of postoperative days required to initiate and perform activities that maintain life, health, and well-being*

Defining Characteristics

- Difficulty in moving about
- Evidence of interrupted healing of surgical area (e.g., red, indurated, draining, immobilized)
- Fatigue
- Loss of appetite with or without nausea
- Perception that more time is needed to recover
- Postpones resumption of work/employment activities
- Requires help to complete self-care
- Report of pain/discomfort

Related Factors

Extensive surgical procedure
Obesity
Pain
Postoperative surgical site infection

Preoperative expectations
Prolonged surgical procedure

References

Kotiniemi, L.H., Ryhanen, P.T., Valanne, J., Jokela, R., Mustonen, A., & Poukkula, E. (1997). Postoperative symptoms at home following day-care surgery in children: A multicentre survey of 551 children. *Anaesthesia, 52*, 963-969.

Kleinbeck, S.V. (2000). Self-reported at-home postoperative recovery. *Research in Nursing & Health, 23*, 461-472.

Zalon, M. (2004). Correlates of recovery among older adults after major abdominal surgery. *Nursing Research, 53*, 99-106.

S

IMPAIRED SWALLOWING
(1986, 1998)

Definition *Abnormal functioning of the swallowing mechanism associated with deficits in oral, pharyngeal, or esophageal structure or function*

Defining Characteristics

Esophageal Phase Impairment

- Abnormality in esophageal phase by swallow study
- Acidic smelling breath
- Bruxism
- Complaints of "something stuck"
- Epigastric pain
- Food refusal
- Heartburn or epigastric pain
- Hematemesis
- Hyperextension of head (e.g., arching during or after meals)
- Nighttime awakening
- Nighttime coughing
- Observed evidence of difficulty in swallowing (e.g., stasis of food in oral cavity, coughing/choking)
- Odynophagia
- Regurgitation of gastric contents (wet burps)
- Repetitive swallowing
- Unexplained irritability surrounding mealtime

- Volume limiting
- Vomiting
- Vomitus on pillow

Oral Phase Impairment

- Abnormality in oral phase of swallow study
- Choking before a swallow
- Coughing before a swallow
- Drooling
- Food falls from mouth
- Food pushed out of mouth
- Gagging before a swallow
- Inability to clear oral cavity
- Incomplete lip closure
- Lack of chewing
- Lack of tongue action to form bolus
- Long meals with little consumption
- Nasal reflux
- Piecemeal deglutition
- Pooling in lateral sulci
- Premature entry of bolus
- Sialorrhea
- Slow bolus formation

S

- Weak suck resulting in inefficient nippling

Pharyngeal Phase Impairment

- Abnormality in pharyngeal phase by swallow study
- Altered head positions
- Choking
- Coughing
- Delayed swallow
- Food refusal
- Gagging
- Gurgly voice quality
- Inadequate laryngeal elevation
- Multiple swallows
- Nasal reflux
- Recurrent pulmonary infections
- Unexplained fevers

Related Factors
Congenital Deficits

Behavioral feeding problems
Conditions with significant hypotonia
Congenital heart disease
Failure to thrive
History of tube feeding
Mechanical obstruction (e.g., edema, tracheostomy tube, tumor)
Neuromuscular impairment (e.g., decreased or absent gag reflex, decreased strength or excursion of muscles involved in mastication, perceptual impairment, facial paralysis)
Protein energy malnutrition
Respiratory disorders
Self-injurious behavior
Upper airway anomalies

Neurological Problems

Achalasia
Acquired anatomic defects
Cerebral palsy
Cranial nerve involvement
Developmental delay
Esophageal defects
Gastroesophageal reflux disease
Laryngeal abnormalities
Laryngeal defects
Nasal defects
Nasopharyngeal cavity defects
Oropharynx abnormalities
Prematurity
Tracheal defects
Traumas
Traumatic head injury
Upper airway anomalies

EFFECTIVE THERAPEUTIC REGIMEN MANAGEMENT
(1994)

Definition *Pattern of regulating and integrating into daily living a program for treatment of illness and its sequelae that is satisfactory for meeting specific health goals*

Defining Characteristics

- Appropriate choices of daily activities for meeting the goals of a prevention program
- Appropriate choices of daily activities for meeting the goals of a treatment program
- Illness symptoms within a normal range of expectation
- Verbalizes desire to manage the treatment of illness
- Verbalizes desire to manage prevention of sequelae
- Verbalizes intent to reduce risk factors for progression of illness and sequelae

Related Factors

To be developed

Note. This diagnosis will retire from the NANDA-I Taxonomy in the 2009–2010 edition unless additional work is done to bring it to a LOE of 2.1 or higher.

INEFFECTIVE THERAPEUTIC REGIMEN MANAGEMENT
(1992)

Definition *Pattern of regulating and integrating into daily living a program for treatment of illness and the sequelae of illness that is unsatisfactory for meeting specific health goals*

Defining Characteristics

- Failure to include treatment regimens in daily routines
- Failure to take action to reduce risk factors
- Makes choices in daily living ineffective for meeting health goals
- Verbalizes desire to manage the illness
- Verbalizes difficulty with prescribed regimens

Related Factors

Complexity of healthcare system
Complexity of therapeutic regimen
Decisional conflicts
Economic difficulties
Excessive demands made (e.g., individual, family)
Family conflict
Family patterns of health care
Inadequate number of cues to action

Knowledge deficit
Mistrust of healthcare personnel
Mistrust of regimen
Perceived barriers
Powerlessness
Perceived seriousness
Perceived susceptibility
Perceived benefits
Social support deficit

INEFFECTIVE COMMUNITY THERAPEUTIC REGIMEN MANAGEMENT
(1994)

Definition *Pattern of regulating and integrating into community processes programs for treatment of illness and the sequelae of illness that are unsatisfactory for meeting health-related goals*

Defining Characteristics

- Deficits in advocates for aggregates
- Deficits in community activities for prevention
- Illness symptoms above the norm expected for the population
- Insufficient healthcare resources (e.g., people, programs)
- Unavailable healthcare resources for illness care
- Unexpected acceleration of illness

Related Factors

To be developed

T

Note. This diagnosis will retire from the NANDA-I Taxonomy in the 2009–2010 edition unless additional work is done to bring it to a LOE of 2.1 or higher.

INEFFECTIVE FAMILY THERAPEUTIC REGIMEN MANAGEMENT
(1994)

Definition *Pattern of regulating and integrating into family processes a program for treatment of illness and the sequelae of illness that is unsatisfactory for meeting specific health goals*

Defining Characteristics

- Acceleration of illness symptoms of a family member
- Inappropriate family activities for meeting health goals
- Failure to take action to reduce risk factors
- Lack of attention to illness
- Verbalizes desire to manage the illness
- Verbalizes difficulty with therapeutic regimen

Related Factors

Complexity of healthcare system
Complexity of therapeutic regimen
Decisional conflicts
Economic difficulties
Excessive demands
Family conflict

READINESS FOR ENHANCED
Therapeutic Regimen Management
(2002, LOE 2.1)

Definition *A pattern of regulating and integrating into daily living a program for treatment of illness and its sequelae that is sufficient for meeting health-related goals and can be strengthened*

Defining Characteristics
- Choices of daily living are appropriate for meeting goals (e.g., treatment, prevention)
- Describes reduction of risk factors
- Expresses desire to manage the illness (e.g., treatment, prevention of sequelae)
- Expresses little difficulty with prescribed regimens
- No unexpected acceleration of illness symptoms

T

INEFFECTIVE **T**HERMOREGULATION
(1986)

Definition *Temperature fluctuation between hypothermia and hyperthermia*

Defining Characteristics

- Cool skin
- Cyanotic nail beds
- Fluctuations in body temperature above and below the normal range
- Flushed skin
- Hypertension
- Increased respiratory rate
- Mild shivering
- Moderate pallor
- Piloerection
- Reduction in body temperature below normal range
- Seizures
- Slow capillary refill
- Tachycardia
- Warm to touch

Related Factors

Aging
Fluctuating environmental
  temperature
Illness
Immaturity
Trauma

DISTURBED THOUGHT PROCESSES
(1973, 1996)

Definition   *Disruption in cognitive operations and activities*

Defining Characteristics
- Cognitive dissonance
- Distractibility
- Egocentricity
- Hypervigilance
- Hypovigilance
- Inaccurate interpretation of environment
- Inappropriate thinking
- Memory deficit

Related Factors
To be developed

T

Note.   This diagnosis will retire from the NANDA-I Taxonomy in the 2009–2010 edition unless additional work is done to bring it to a LOE of 2.1 or higher.

IMPAIRED TISSUE INTEGRITY
(1986, 1998)

Definition   *Damage to mucous membrane, corneal, integumentary, or subcutaneous tissues*

Defining Characteristics

- Damaged tissue (e.g., cornea, mucous membrane, integumentary, subcutaneous)
- Destroyed tissue

Related Factors

Altered circulation
Chemical irritants
Fluid deficit
Fluid excess
Impaired physical mobility
Knowledge deficit

Mechanical factors (e.g., pressure, shear, friction)
Nutritional factors (e.g., deficit or excess)
Radiation
Temperature extremes

INEFFECTIVE TISSUE PERFUSION (Specify Type: Renal, Cerebral, Cardiopulmonary, Gastrointestinal, Peripheral)
(1980, 1998)

Definition *Decrease in oxygen resulting in the failure to nourish the tissues at the capillary level*

Defining Characteristics

Cardiopulmonary
- Abnormal arterial blood gases
- Altered respiratory rate outside of acceptable parameters
- Arrhythmias
- Bronchospasm
- Capillary refill > 3 seconds
- Chest pain
- Chest retraction
- Dyspnea
- Nasal flaring
- Sense of "impending doom"
- Use of accessory muscles

Cerebral
- Altered mental status
- Behavioral changes
- Changes in motor response
- Changes in pupillary reactions
- Difficulty in swallowing
- Extremity weakness
- Paralysis

- Speech abnormalities

Gastrointestinal
- Abdominal distention
- Abdominal pain or tenderness
- Absent bowel sounds
- Hypoactive bowel sounds
- Nausea

Peripheral
- Absent pulses
- Altered sensations
- Altered skin characteristics (e.g., hair, nails, moisture)
- Blood pressure changes in extremities
- Bruits
- Claudication
- Delayed healing
- Diminished arterial pulsations
- Edema
- Positive Homan's sign
- Skin color pales on elevation; color does not return on lowering the leg

- Skin discolorations
- Skin temperature changes
- Weak pulses

  Renal

- Altered blood pressure outside of acceptable parameters
- Anuria

- Elevation in BUN/creatinine ratio
- Hematuria
- Oliguria

Related Factors

Altered affinity of hemoglobin for oxygen
Decreased hemoglobin concentration in blood
Enzyme poisoning
Exchange problems
Hypoventilation

Hypovolemia
Hypervolemia
Impaired transport of oxygen
Interruption of blood flow
Mismatch of ventilation with blood flow

T

IMPAIRED TRANSFER ABILITY
(1998, 2006, LOE 2.1)

Definition *Limitation of independent movement between two nearby surfaces*

Defining Characteristics
- Inability to transfer between uneven levels
- Inability to transfer from bed to chair
- Inability to transfer from chair to bed
- Inability to transfer on or off a toilet
- Inability to transfer on or off a commode
- Inability to transfer in or out of tub
- Inability to transfer in or out of shower
- Inability to transfer from chair to car
- Inability to transfer from car to chair
- Inability to transfer from chair to floor
- Inability to transfer from floor to chair
- Inability to transfer from standing to floor
- Inability to transfer from floor to standing
- Inability to transfer from bed to standing
- Inability to transfer from standing to bed
- Inability to transfer from chair to standing
- Inability to transfer from standing to chair

Related Factors
Insufficient muscle strength
Neuromuscular impairment
Musculoskeletal impairment (e.g., contractures)

Pain
Cognitive impairment
Obesity

Note. Specify level of independence using a standardized functional scale.

Environmental constraints (e.g., bed height, inadequate space, wheel chair type, treatment equipment, restraints)

Lack of knowledge
Impaired balance
Deconditioning
Impaired vision

References

Brouwer, K., Nysseknabm, J., & Culham E. (2004). Physical function and health status among seniors with and without fear of falling. *Gerontology, 50,* 15-141.

Lewis, C.L., Moutoux, M., Slaughter, M., & Bailey, S.P. (2004). Characteristics of individuals who fell while receiving home health services. *Physical Therapy,* 84(1), 23-32.

Tinetti., M.E., & Ginter, S.F. (1988). Identifying mobility dysfunction in elderly persons. *Journal of American Medical Association, 259,* 1190-1193.

RISK FOR TRAUMA
(1980)

Definition *Accentuated risk of accidental tissue injury (e.g., wound, burn, fracture)*

Risk Factors
External
Accessability of guns

Bathing in very hot water (e.g., unsupervised bathing of young children)

Bathtub without antislip equipment

Children playing with dangerous objects

Children playing without gates at top of stairs

Children riding in the front seat in car

Contact with corrosives

Contact with intense cold

Contact with rapidly moving machinery

Defective appliances

Delayed lighting of gas appliances

Driving a mechanically unsafe vehicle

Driving at excessive speeds

Driving while intoxicated

Driving without necessary visual aids

Entering unlighted rooms

Experimenting with chemicals

Exposure to dangerous machinery

Faulty electrical plugs

Flammable children's clothing

Flammable children's toys

Frayed wires

Grease waste collected on stoves

High beds

High-crime neighborhood

Inappropriate call-for-aid mechanisms for bed-resting client

Inadequate stair rails

Inadequately stored combustibles (e.g., matches, oily rags)

Inadequately stored corrosives (e.g., lye)

Knives stored uncovered

Lack of protection from heat source

Large icicles hanging from the roof

Misuse of necessary headgear
Misuse of seat restraints
Nonuse of seat restraints
Obstructed passageways
Overexposure to radiation
Overloaded electrical outlets
Overloaded fuse boxes
Physical proximity to vehicle pathways (e.g., driveways, lanes, railroad tracks)
Playing with explosives
Pot handles facing toward front of stove
Potential igniting of gas leaks
Slippery floors (e.g., wet or highly waxed)
Smoking in bed
Smoking near oxygen
Struggling with restraints
Unanchored electric wires
Unanchored rugs
Unsafe road
Unsafe walkways
Unsafe window protection in homes with young children
Use of cracked dishware
Use of unsteady chairs
Use of unsteady ladders
Wearing flowing clothes around open flame

Internal

Balancing difficulties
Cognitive difficulties
Emotional difficulties
History of previous trauma
Insufficient finances
Lack of safety education
Lack of safety precautions
Poor vision
Reduced hand-eye coordination
Reduced muscle coordination
Reduced sensation
Weakness

IMPAIRED URINARY ELIMINATION
(1973, 2006, LOE 2.1)

Definition *Dysfunction in urine elimination*

Defining Characteristics
- Dysuria
- Frequency
- Hesitancy
- Incontinence
- Nocturia
- Retention
- Urgency

Related Factors
Anatomical obstruction
Multiple causality
Sensory motor impair-
    ment
Urinary tract infection

References

Engberg, S., McDowell, B., Donovan, N., Brodak, I., & Weber, E. (1997). Treatment of urinary incontinence in homebound older adults: Interface between research and practice. *Ostomy/Wound Management, 48*(10), 18-26.

Fantl, J., Newman, D., & Colling, J. (1996). *Urinary incontinence in adults: Acute and chronic management* (clinical practice guideline No. 2). Rockville, MD: U.S. Department of Health & Human Services.

Messick, G., & Powe, C. (1997). Applying behavioral research to incontinence. *Ostomy/Wound Management, 48*(10), 40-48.

READINESS FOR ENHANCED URINARY ELIMINATION
(2002, LOE 2.1)

Definition *A pattern of urinary functions that is sufficient for meeting eliminatory needs and can be strengthened*

Defining Characteristics

- Amount of output is within normal limits
- Expresses willingness to enhance urinary elimination
- Fluid intake is adequate for daily needs
- Positions self for emptying of bladder
- Specific gravity is within normal limits
- Urine is odorless
- Urine is straw colored

U

URINARY RETENTION
(1986)

Definition *Incomplete emptying of the bladder*

Defining Characteristics

- Absence of urine output
- Bladder distention
- Dribbling
- Dysuria
- Frequent voiding
- Overflow incontinence
- Residual urine
- Sensation of bladder fullness
- Small voiding

Related Factors

Blockage
High urethral pressure
Inhibition of reflex arc
Strong sphincter

IMPAIRED SPONTANEOUS VENTILATION
(1992)

Definition   *Decreased energy reserves result in an individual's inability to maintain breathing adequate to support life*

Defining Characteristics

- Apprehension
- Decreased cooperation
- Decreased pO2
- Decreased SaO2
- Decreased tidal volume
- Dyspnea
- Increased heart rate
- Increased metabolic rate
- Increased pCO2
- Increased restlessness
- Increased use of accessory muscles

Related Factors

Metabolic factors
Respiratory muscle fatigue

V

DYSFUNCTIONAL VENTILATORY WEANING RESPONSE
(1992)

Definition *Inability to adjust to lowered levels of mechanical ventilator support that interrupts and prolongs the weaning process*

Defining Characteristics

Mild

- Breathing discomfort
- Expressed feelings of increased need for oxygen
- Fatigue
- Increased concentration on breathing
- Queries about possible machine malfunction
- Restlessness
- Slight increase of respiratory rate from baseline
- Warmth

Moderate

- Apprehension
- Baseline increase in respiratory rate (<5 breaths/min)
- Color changes
- Decreased air entry on auscultation
- Diaphoresis
- Hypervigilance to activities
- Inability to cooperate
- Inability to respond to coaching

- Pale
- Slight cyanosis
- Slight increase from baseline blood pressure (<20 mm Hg)
- Slight increase from baseline heart rate (<20 beats/ min)
- Slight respiratory accessory muscle use
- Wide-eyed look

Severe

- Adventitious breath sounds
- Agitation
- Asynchronized breathing with the ventilator
- Audible airway secretions
- Cyanosis
- Decreased level of consciousness
- Deterioration in arterial blood gases from current baseline
- Full respiratory accessory muscle use
- Gasping breaths

V

- Increase from baseline blood pressure (≥20 mm Hg)
- Increase from baseline heart rate (≥20 breaths/min)

- Paradoxical abdominal breathing
- Profuse diaphoresis
- Respiratory rate increases significantly from baseline
- Shallow breaths

Related Factors

Physiological

Inadequate nutrition
Ineffective airway clearance
Sleep pattern disturbance
Uncontrolled pain

Psychological

Anxiety
Decreased motivation
Decreased self-esteem
Fear
Hopelessness
Insufficient trust in the nurse
Knowledge deficit of the weaning process
Patient perceived inefficacy about ability to wean
Powerlessness

Situational

Adverse environment (e.g., noisy, active environment; negative events in the room, low nurse-patient ratio, unfamiliar nursing staff)
History of multiple unsuccessful weaning attempts
History of ventilator dependence >4 days
Inadequate social support
Inappropriate pacing of diminished ventilator support
Uncontrolled episodic energy demands

V

RISK FOR OTHER-DIRECTED VIOLENCE
(1980, 1996)

Definition *At risk for behaviors in which an individual demonstrates that he/she can be physically, emotionally, and/or sexually harmful to others*

Risk Factors

Availability of weapon(s)
Body language (e.g., rigid posture, clenching of fists and jaw, hyperactivity, pacing, breathlessness, threatening stances)
Cognitive impairment (e.g., learning disabilities, attention deficit disorder, decreased intellectual functioning)
Cruelty to animals
Firesetting
History of childhood abuse
History of indirect violence (e.g., tearing off clothes, ripping objects off walls, writing on walls, urinating on floor, defecating on floor, stamping feet, temper tantrum, running in corridors, yelling, throwing objects, breaking a window, slamming doors, sexual advances)
History of substance abuse
History of threats of violence (e.g., verbal threats against property, verbal threats against person, social threats, cursing, threatening notes/letters, threatening gestures, sexual threats)
History of witnessing family violence
History of violence against others (e.g., hitting someone, kicking someone, spitting at someone, scratching someone, throwing objects at someone, biting someone, attempted rape, rape, sexual molestation, urinating/defecating on a person)

V

History of violent antisocial behavior (e.g., stealing, insistent borrowing, insistent demands for privileges, insistent interruption of meetings, refusal to eat, refusal to take medication, ignoring instructions)

Impulsivity

Motor vehicle offenses (e.g., frequent traffic violations, use of a motor vehicle to release anger)

Neurological impairment (e.g., positive EEG, CAT, MRI, neurological findings; head trauma; seizure disorders)

Pathological intoxication

Perinatal complications

Prenatal complications

Psychotic symptomatology (e.g., auditory, visual, command hallucinations; paranoid delusions; loose, rambling, or illogical thought processes)

Suicidal behavior

V

RISK FOR SELF-DIRECTED VIOLENCE
(1994)

Definition *At risk for behaviors in which an individual demonstrates that he/she can be physically, emotionally and/or sexually harmful to self*

Risk Factors

Age 15 - 19

Age over 45

Behavioral clues (e.g., writing forlorn love notes, directing angry messages at a significant other who has rejected the person, giving away personal items, taking out a large life insurance policy)

Conflictual interpersonal relationships

Emotional problems (e.g., hopelessness, despair, increased anxiety, panic, anger, hostility)

Employment problems (e.g., unemployed, recent job loss/ failure)

Engagement in autoerotic sexual acts

Family background (e.g., chaotic or conflictual, history of suicide)

History of multiple suicide attempts

Lack of personal resources (e.g., poor achievement, poor insight, affect unavailable and poorly controlled)

Lack of social resources (e.g., poor rapport, socially isolated, unresponsive family)

Physical health problems (e.g., hypochondriasis, chronic or terminal illness)

Marital status (single, widowed, divorced)

Mental health problems (e.g., severe depression, psychosis, severe personality disorder, alcoholism or drug abuse)

Occupation (executive, administrator/owner of business, professional, semiskilled worker)

Sexual orientation (bisexual [active], homosexual [inactive])

Suicidal ideation

V

Suicidal plan
Verbal clues (e.g., talking
   about death, "better off
   without me," asking
   questions about lethal
   dosages of drugs)

V

IMPAIRED **W**ALKING
(1998, 2006, LOE 2.1)

Definition *Limitation of independent movement within the environment on foot*

Defining Characteristics
- Impaired ability to climb stairs
- Impaired ability to navigate curbs
- Impaired ability to walk required distances
- Impaired ability to walk on incline
- Impaired ability to walk on decline
- Impaired ability to walk on uneven surfaces

Risk Factors

Cognitive impairment
Deconditioning
Depressed mood
Environmental constraints (e.g., stairs, inclines, uneven surfaces, unsafe obstacles, distances, lack of assistive devices or person, restraints)
Fear of falling
Impaired balance

Impaired vision
Insufficient muscle strength
Lack of knowledge
Limited endurance
Musculoskeletal impairment (e.g., contractures)
Neuromuscular impairment
Obesity
Pain

Note. Specify level of independence using a standardized functional scale.

W

References

Brouwer, K., Nysseknabm, J., & Culham E. (2004). Physical function and health status among seniors with and without fear of falling. *Gerontology, 50,* 15-141.

Lewis, C.L., Moutoux, M., Slaughter, M., & Bailey, S.P. (2004). Characteristics of individuals who fell while receiving home health services. *Physical Therapy,* 84(1), 23-32.

Tinetti, M.E., & Ginter, S.F. (1988). Identifying mobility dysfunction in elderly persons. *Journal of American Medical Association, 259,* 1190-1193.

W

WANDERING
(2000)

Definition   *Meandering, aimless or repetitive locomotion that exposes the individual to harm; frequently incongruent with boundaries, limits, or obstacles*

Defining Characteristics

- Continuous movement from place to place
- Getting lost
- Fretful locomotion
- Frequent movement from place to place
- Haphazard locomotion
- Hyperactivity
- Inability to locate significant landmarks in a familiar setting
- Locomotion into unauthorized or private spaces
- Locomotion resulting in unintended leaving of a premise
- Locomotion that cannot be easily dissuaded
- Long periods of locomotion without an apparent destination
- Pacing
- Periods of locomotion interspersed with periods of nonlocomotion (e.g., sitting, standing, sleeping)
- Persistent locomotion in search of something
- Shadowing a caregiver's locomotion
- Trespassing
- Scanning behaviors
- Searching behaviors

Related Factors

Cognitive impairment (e.g., memory and recall deficits, disorientation, poor visuoconstructive or visuospatial ability, language defects)

Cortical atrophy
Emotional state (e.g., frustration, anxiety, boredom, depression, agitation)
Overstimulating environment

W

Physiological state or need (e.g., hunger, thirst, pain, urination, constipation)

Premorbid behavior (e.g., outgoing, sociable personality; premorbid dementia)

Sedation

Separation from familiar environment

Time of day

W

Part 2

TAXONOMY II

2007–2008

Part 2 describes the historical development and structure of Taxonomy II. It includes a discussion of the
multiaxial structure of the taxonomy with its three levels:
Domains, Classes, and Nursing Diagnoses; the future
mapping of the nursing diagnoses in the NANDA, NIC and
NOC (NNN) Common Structure; and the NNN Taxonomy
of Nursing Practice.

History of the Development of Taxonomy II

Following the biennial conference in April 1994, the Taxonomy Committee met to place newly submitted diagnoses
into the Taxonomy I revised structure. The committee had
considerable difficulty, however, categorizing some of these
diagnoses. Given this difficulty and the expanding number
of submissions at level 1.4 and higher, the committee felt a
new taxonomic structure was necessary. This possibility
gave rise to considerable discussion as to how this might be
accomplished.

To begin, the committee agreed to determine if there were
categories that arose naturally from the data, i.e., from
accepted diagnoses. Round One of a naturalistic Q sort
was completed later at the 11th biennial conference in 1994
in Nashville, Tennessee. Round Two was completed later
and the analysis presented at the 12th biennial conference in
1996 in Pittsburgh, Pennsylvania. That Q sort yielded 21 categories, far too many to be useful or practical.

In 1998, the Taxonomy Committee sent four Q sorts using
four different frameworks to the NANDA Board of Directors. Framework One, reported in 1996, was in the naturalistic style. Framework Two used Jenny's (1994) ideas. Framework Three used the Nursing Outcomes Classifications
(NOC) (Johnson & Maas, 1997), and Framework Four used
Gordon's (1998) Functional Health Patterns. No one of these
was entirely satisfactory, although Gordon's was the best fit.
With Gordon's permission, the Taxonomy Committee
slightly modified her framework to create Framework Five,
which was presented to the membership in April 1998 at the

13th biennial conference in St. Louis, Missouri. At that conference, the Taxonomy Committee invited the members to sort the diagnoses according to domains that had been selected. By the end of the conference, 40 usable sets of data were available for analysis. During the data collection phase at the conference, members of the Taxonomy Committee took careful notes of the questions asked, the confusion expressed by members, and the suggestions for improvements.

Based on the analysis of the data and the field notes, additional modifications were made to the framework. One domain of the original framework was divided into two to reduce the number of classes and diagnoses falling within it. A separate domain was added for growth and development since the original framework did not contain that domain. Several other domains were renamed to better reflect the content of the diagnoses within them. The final taxonomic structure is much less like Gordon's original, but has reduced misclassification errors and redundancies to near zero, which is a much desired state in a taxonomic structure.

Finally, definitions were developed for all the domains and classes within the structure. The definition of each diagnosis was then compared to that of the class and the domain in which it was placed. Revisions and modifications in the diagnosis placements were made to ensure maximum match among domain, class, and diagnosis.

In 2002, following the NANDA, NIC, & NOC (NNN) Conference in Chicago, the approved nursing diagnoses were placed in Taxonomy II. These included 11 health promotion nursing diagnoses as well as the revised and newly approved nursing diagnoses. In the future, as new nursing diagnoses are developed and approved, they will be added to the taxonomic structure in the appropriate locations. In January 2003, the Taxonomy Committee met in Chicago and made further refinements to the terminology in Taxonomy II. Following the 2004 NNN Conference in Chicago, the Taxonomy Committee placed the newly approved nursing diagnoses in their appropriate categories. The Taxonomy Committee, to foster its international focus, reviewed the axes in Taxonomy II and compared them to the International Standards Organization (ISO) Reference Terminology Model for a Nursing Diagnosis.

Structure of Taxonomy II

Clinicians are primarily concerned with the diagnoses within the taxonomy and rarely need to use the taxonomic structure itself. Familiarity with how a diagnosis is structured, however, will aid the clinician who needs to find information quickly and those who wish to submit new diagnoses. A brief explanation of how the taxonomy is designed is therefore included here.

Taxonomy II has three levels: domains, classes, and nursing diagnoses. Figure 2.1 (page 266) depicts the organization of domains and classes in Taxonomy II. Some nursing diagnoses lend themselves to placement in more than one domain and class. This occurs because the nursing diagnosis label, definition, defining characteristics or related factors—in the instance of "risk for"—lend themselves to appropriate location in more than one domain and class.

Table 2.1 (page 271) shows Taxonomy II with 13 domains, 47 classes, and 188 diagnoses. A domain is "a sphere of activity, study or interest" (Roget, 1980, p. 287). A class is "a subdivision of a larger group; a division of persons or things by quality, rank, or grade" (Roget, p. 157). "A nursing diagnosis is a clinical judgment about an individual, family or community response to actual or potential health problems/life processes which provides the basis for definitive therapy toward achievement of outcomes for which a nurse is accountable" (see p. 332)

The Taxonomy II code structure is a 32-bit integer (or if the user's database uses another notation, the code structure is a 5-digit code). This structure provides for the growth and development of the classification structure without having to change codes when new diagnoses, refinements, and revisions are added. New codes are assigned to the nursing diagnoses when they are approved by the Board of Directors upon the recommendation of the Diagnosis Development Committee, following an open forum hearing at the biennial conference.

Taxonomy II has a code structure that is compliant with recommendations from the National Library of Medicine (NLM) concerning healthcare terminology codes. The NLM recommends that codes not contain information about the classified concept, as did the Taxonomy I code structure, which included information about the location and the level of the diagnosis.

The NANDA-I Taxonomy is a recognized nursing language that meets the criteria established by the Committee for Nursing Practice Information Infrastructure (CNPII) of the American Nurses Association (ANA) (Coenen, McNeil, Bakken, Bickford, & Warren, 2001). The benefit of being included as a recognized nursing language indicates that the classification system is accepted as supporting nursing practice by providing clinically useful terminology. The ANA recognition facilitates the inclusion of NANDA-I in the ANA Nursing Information and Data Set Evaluation Center (NIDSEC) criteria for clinical information systems (nursingworld.org/nidsec/index.htm) and the National Library of Medicine's (NLM's) Unified Medical Language System (UMLS) (www.nlm.nih.gov/research/umls/umlsmain.html). The taxonomy is registered with Health Level Seven (HL7), a healthcare informatics standard, as a terminology to be used in identifying nursing diagnoses in electronic messages among clinical information systems (www.HL7.org). NANDA-I diagnoses have been modeled into SNOMED CT, which has been accepted as a terminology standard for the United States Department of Health and Human Services, the United States Consolidated Health Information Initiative, and the United Kingdom's National Health Service. A map of this modeling effort is available from SNOMED International (www.snomed.org).

The NANDA-I Taxonomy nursing diagnoses also comply with the International Standards Organization (ISO) terminology model for a nursing diagnosis (Figure 2.2, page 268).

The Multiaxial System

Taxonomy II is multiaxial in form. This format substantially improves the flexibility of the nomenclature and allows for easy additions and modifications.

An axis, for the purpose of the NANDA-I Taxonomy, is operationally defined as a dimension of the human response that is considered in the diagnostic process.

There are seven axes. The NANDA-I Model of a Nursing Diagnosis displays the seven axes and their relationship to one another (Figure 2.3, page 268). The ordering and some of the labels and definitions have been changed since the 2005-2006 edition of this book in order to parallel the International Standards Reference Model for a Nursing Diagnosis.

Axis 1 The diagnostic concept
Axis 2 Subject of the diagnosis (individual, family, community)
Axis 3 Judgment (impaired, ineffective)
Axis 4 Location (bladder, auditory, cerebral)
Axis 5 Age (infant, child, adult)
Axis 6 Time (chronic, acute, intermittent)
Axis 7 Status of the diagnosis (actual, risk, wellness, health promotion)

The axes are represented in the named/coded nursing diagnoses through their values. In some cases, they are named explicitly — e.g., *ineffective community coping* and *compromised family coping*—in which the subject of the diagnosis (in the first instance "community" and in the second instance "family") is named using the two values "community" and "family" taken from Axis 2 (subject of the diagnosis). "Ineffective" and "compromised" are two of the values contained in Axis 3 (judgment).

In some cases, the axis is implicit — e.g., *activity tolerance* — in which the subject of the diagnosis (Axis 2) is always the individual. In some instances an axis may not be pertinent to a particular diagnosis and therefore not part of the nursing diagnostic label or code. For example, the time axis may not be relevant to every diagnosis.

Axis 1 (the diagnostic concept) and Axis 3 (judgment) are essential components of a nursing diagnosis. In some cases, however, the diagnostic concept contains the judgment (e.g., *pain*); in these cases the judgment is not explicitly separated out in the diagnostic label. Axis 2 (subject of the diagnosis) is also essential, although, as described above, it may be implied and therefore not included in the label. The Diagnostic Development Committee require these axes for submission; the other axes may be used where relevant for clarity.

Definitions of the Axes
Axis 1 The Diagnostic Concept

The diagnostic concept is the principal element or the fundamental and essential part, the root, of the diagnostic statement. It describes the "human response" that is the core of the diagnosis.

The diagnostic concept may consist of one or more nouns. When more than one noun is used (e.g., *activity tolerance*), each one contributes a unique meaning to the concept, as if the two were a single noun; the meaning of the combined term, however, is different from when the nouns are stated separately. Frequently, an adjective (e.g., spiritual) may be used with a noun (e.g., distress) to denote the diagnostic concept *spiritual distress*.

In some cases, the diagnostic concept and the diagnosis are one and the same, e.g., *pain*. This occurs when the nursing diagnosis is stated at its most clinically useful level and the separation of the diagnostic concept adds no meaningful level of abstraction.

The diagnostic concepts in Taxonomy II are:

- Activity intolerance
- Adaptive capacity
- Airway clearance
- Anxiety
- Aspiration
- Attachment
- Autonomic dysreflexia
- Bathing/hygiene self-care
- Bed mobility
- Body image
- Body temperature
- Breastfeeding
- Breathing pattern
- Cardiac output

- Caregiver role strain
- Communication
- Comfort
- Confusion
- Constipation
- Contamination
- Coping
- Death anxiety
- Decisional conflict
- Denial
- Dentition
- Development
- Diarrhea
- Disuse syndrome
- Diversional activity
- Dressing/grooming self-care
- Dysreflexia
- Elimination
- Energy field
- Environmental interpretation
- Failure to thrive
- Falls
- Family processes
- Family processes: Alcoholism
- Fatigue
- Fear
- Feeding self-care
- Fluid balance
- Fluid volume
- Functional incontinence
- Gas exchange
- Glucose level
- Grieving
- Growth
- Health maintenance
- Health-seeking behaviors
- Home maintenance
- Hope
- Hopelessness
- Human dignity
- Hyperthermia
- Hypothermia
- Identity
- Immunization status
- Incontinence
- Infant behavior
- Infant feeding pattern
- Infection
- Injury
- Insomnia
- Intracranial adaptive behavior
- Knowledge
- Latex allergy response
- Liver function
- Loneliness
- Memory
- Mobility
- Moral distress
- Mucous membrane
- Nausea
- Neurovascular function
- Noncompliance
- Nutrition
- Other-directed violence
- Pain
- Parent/child attachment
- Parental role conflict
- Parenting
- Perioperative-positioning injury
- Peripheral neurovascular dysfunction

- Physical mobility
- Poisoning
- Post-trauma syndrome
- Power
- Powerlessness
- Protection
- Rape-trauma syndrome
- Rape-trauma compound reaction
- Rape-trauma silent reaction
- Reflex incontinence
- Religiosity
- Relocation stress syndrome
- Retention
- Risk-prone health behavior
- Role conflict
- Role performance
- Sedentary lifestyle
- Self-care
- Self-care deficit
- Self-concept
- Self-directed violence
- Self-esteem
- Self-mutilation
- Sensory perception
- Sexual dysfunction
- Sexual function
- Sexuality patterns
- Skin integrity
- Sleep
- Sleep deprivation
- Sleep pattern
- Social interaction
- Social isolation
- Sorrow
- Spiritual distress
- Spiritual well-being
- Spontaneous ventilation
- Stress incontinence
- Stress overload
- Sudden infant death syndrome
- Suicide
- Suffocation
- Surgical recovery
- Swallowing
- Therapeutic regimen management
- Thermoregulation
- Thought process
- Tissue integrity
- Tissue perfusion
- Toileting self-care
- Total incontinence
- Transfer
- Transfer ability
- Trauma
- Unilateral neglect
- Urge incontinence
- Urinary elimination
- Urinary retention
- Ventilatory weaning response
- Verbal communication
- Violence
- Walking
- Wandering
- Wheelchair mobility

Axis 2 Subject of the Diagnosis

The subject of the diagnosis is defined as the person(s) for whom a nursing diagnosis is determined. The values in Axis 2 are individual, family, group, and community:

- *Individual:* A single human being distinct from others, a person
- *Family:* Two or more people having continuous or sustained relationships, perceiving reciprocal obligations, sensing common meaning, and sharing certain obligations toward others; related by blood and/or choice
- *Group:* A number of people with shared characteristics
- *Community:* A group of people living in the same locale under the same governance. Examples include neighborhoods and cities.

When the subject of the diagnosis is not explicitly stated, it becomes the individual by default.

Axis 3 Judgment

A judgment is a descriptor or modifier that limits or specifies the meaning of the diagnostic concept. The diagnostic concept together with the nurse's judgment about it forms the diagnosis. The values in Axis 3 are:

Value	Definition
• Anticipatory	Realize beforehand, foresee
• Compromised	Damaged, made vulnerable
• Decreased	Lessened (in size, amount, or degree)
• Defensive	Used or intended to defend or protect
• Deficient	Insufficient, inadequate
• Delayed	Late, slow, or postponed
• Disabled	Limited, handicapped
• Disorganized	Not properly arranged or controlled
• Disproportionate	Too large or too small in comparison with norm

- Disturbed — Agitated, interrupted, interfered with
- Dysfunctional — Not operating normally
- Effective — Producing the intended or desired effect
- Enhanced — Improved in quality, value, or extent
- Excessive — Greater than necessary or desirable
- Imbalanced — Out of proportion or balance
- Impaired — Damaged, weakened
- Ineffective — Not producing the intended or desired effect
- Interrupted — Having its continuity broken
- Low — Below the norm
- Organized — Properly arranged or controlled
- Perceived — Observed through the senses
- Readiness for — In a suitable state for an activity or situation
- Situational — Related to a particular circumstance

Axis 4 Location

Location describes the parts/regions of the body and/or their related functions–all tissues, organs, anatomical sites, or structures. The values in Axis 4 are:

- Auditory
- Bladder
- Cardiopulmonary
- Cerebral
- Gastrointestinal
- Gustatory
- Intracranial
- Kinesthetic
- Mucous membranes
- Oral
- Olfactory
- Peripheral neurovascular
- Peripheral vascular
- Renal
- Skin
- Tactile
- Visual

Axis 5 Age

Age refers to the age of the person who is the subject of the diagnosis (Axis 2). The values in Axis 4 are:

- Fetus
- Neonate
- Infant
- Toddler
- Preschool child

- School-age child
- Adolescent
- Adult
- Infant
- Older adult

Axis 6 Time

Time describes the duration of the diagnostic concept (Axis 1). The values in Axis 6 are:

- *Acute:* Lasting less than six months
- *Chronic:* Lasting more than six months
- *Intermittent:* Stopping or starting again at intervals, periodic, cyclic
- *Continuous:* Uninterrupted, going on without stop

Axis 7 Status of the Diagnosis

Status of the diagnosis refers to the actuality or potentiality of the problem or to the categorization of the diagnosis as a wellness/health promotion diagnosis. The values in Axis 7 are:

- *Actual:* Existing in fact or reality, existing at the present time
- *Health Promotion:* Behavior motivated by the desire to increase well-being and actualize human health potential (Pender, Murduagh, & Parsons, 2006)
- *Risk:* Vulnerability, especially as a result of exposure to factors that increase the chance of injury or loss
- *Wellness:* The quality or state of being healthy

Construction of a Nursing Diagnostic Statement

A nursing diagnosis is constructed by combining the values from Axis 1 (the diagnostic concept), Axis 2 (subject of the diagnosis), and Axis 3 (judgment) where needed and adding values from the other axes for relevant clarity. Thus you begin with the diagnostic concept (Axis 1) and add the judgment (Axis 3) about it. Remember that these two axes are sometimes combined into a single diagnostic concept, e.g. *pain*. Next, you specify the subject of the diagnosis (Axis 2). If the subject is an "individual," you need not make it explicit (Figure 2.4, page 269). You can then use the remaining axes, if they are appropriate, to add more detail.

For example, if the diagnostic concept (Axis 1) is parenting, you can choose "impaired" or "readiness for enhanced" from the judgment axis (Axis 3). In addition, you have five other axes from which to choose appropriate values. You might choose "individual" from Axis 2 (the subject of the diagnosis), "adolescent" from the age axis (Axis 5), and "risk for" from Axis 7 (status of the diagnosis) to arrive at the diagnosis of *risk for impaired individual parenting: adolescent* (Figure 2.5, page 269). Figure 2.6 (page 270) shows the model for the diagnosis *enhanced coping: family*, an example of a wellness/health promotion nursing diagnosis.

Some words of caution as well as encouragement: Using a multiaxial structure allows diagnoses to be constructed that make no sense (such as *impaired self-care: fetus*). You need to use your common sense and nursing knowledge to construct only those diagnoses that have defining characteristics and are thus appropriate for testing.

The NNN Taxonomy of Nursing Practice

NANDA-I's Taxonomy appeared for the first time in *NANDA Nursing Diagnoses: Definitions & Classifications 2001-2002*. During this period, NANDA began to negotiate an alliance with the Classification Center at the College of Nursing, University of Iowa, Iowa City, Iowa. As a part of that alliance, the possibility of developing a common taxonomic structure was explored. The purposes of a common structure are to make relationships among the three classifications — nursing diagnoses, nursing interventions and nursing outcomes — visible and to facilitate the linkage between the three systems. The possibilities were discussed among members of the NANDA-I Board of Directors and the leadership of the Classification Center.

Dorothy Jones, representing NANDA-I, and Joanne McCloskey Dochterman, representing the Classification Center, developed a proposal to convene an invitational conference. The proposal was funded by the National Library of Medicine, and a three-day meeting was held August, 2001 at the Starved Rock Conference Center in Utica, Illinois. It was attended by 24 experts in standardized nursing language development, testing, and refinement. The goal was to develop a common taxonomic structure for nursing practice, including NANDA (nursing diagnoses), NIC (nursing interventions), NOC (nursing outcomes), with the possibility of inclusion of other languages. A detailed account of the conference, as well as the history and development, can be found in *Unifying Nursing Languages: The Harmonization of NANDA, NIC, and NOC* (Dochterman & Jones, 2003).

The NANDA Taxonomy Committee met in January 2003 to place the nursing diagnoses from the *NANDA Nursing Diagnoses: Definitions and Classifications 2003-2004* into the NNN Taxonomy of Nursing Practice. The committee established rules governing the placement of the nursing diagnoses:

1. The nursing diagnosis *definition and defining characteristics guide* the placement of the nursing diagnosis.
2. When a nursing diagnosis *bridges two or more domains,* the Taxonomy Committee reviews the nursing diagnosis definition and defining characteristics and places it in the domain clinically consistent with that information.
3. Upon review of the definition and defining characteristics of a nursing diagnosis, if it is *clinically consistent with two or more domains,* the nursing diagnosis is placed where the practicing nurse would expect to find it.

4. Some nursing diagnoses *can not be placed* because there is no consensus among the members of the Taxonomy Committee. For example, *deficient diversional activity* and *delayed surgical recovery* were not placed because they could fall in several domains and classes.

5. *"Risk for"* or *"Readiness for Enhanced"* nursing diagnoses are placed in the same domain and class as the actual nursing diagnosis, when one exists.

Table 2.2 (page 282) shows the placement of the 188 current nursing diagnosis approved by NANDA-I in the NNN Taxonomy of Nursing Practice.

Nursing Diagnoses Accepted for Further Development

The following diagnoses are at the level of evidence of 1.4, "accepted for further development," and are included in this publication to encourage further development for future submission.

Chronic low self-esteem
Defensive coping
Disturbed personal identity
Disturbed thought processes
Health-seeking behaviors
Ineffective community therapeutic regimen management
Rape trauma syndrome
Rape trauma syndrome: Compound reaction
Rape trauma syndrome: Silent reaction

Further Development of the NANDA-I Taxonomy

A multiaxial framework allows clinicians to see where there are gaps and/or potentially useful new diagnoses. If you construct a new diagnosis or a set of diagnoses that is useful to your practice, please submit it (them) to NANDA-I so others can share in the discovery. Submission guidelines are on page 320. Submission forms can also be found on the NANDA-I Web site (www.nanda.org) and on the NLINKS Web site (www.nlinks.org). The Diagnostic Development Committee will be glad to help you prepare the submission. For assistance and/or questions, contact the committee chair, Leann Scroggins (scroggins.leann@mayo.edu).

NANDA-I's main office can also be a source of information for preparation of the submission of new or revised nursing diagnoses. The office is at 100 North 20th Street, Philadelphia, PA 19103. Telephone: 800.647.9002 or 215.545.8105, fax: 215.545.8107.

References

Coenen, A., McNeil, B., Bakken, S., Bickford, C., & Warren, J. (2001). Toward comparable nursing data: American Nurses Association criteria for data sets, classification systems, and nomenclatures. *Computers in Nursing, 19,* 240–248.

Dochterman, J.M, & Jones, D. (Eds.) (2003). *Unifying nursing languages: The harmonization of NANDA, NIC, and NOC.* Washington, DC: American Nurses Association.

Gordon. M. (1998). *Manual of nursing diagnosis.* St. Louis: Mosby.

Jenny, J. (1994). Advancing the science of nursing with nursing diagnosis. In M. Rantz & P. LeMone (Eds.), *Classification of nursing diagnoses: Proceedings of the eleventh conference* (pp. 73–81). Glendale, CA: CINAHL.

Johnson, M., & Maas, M. (1997). *Nursing outcomes classification* (NOC). St. Louis: Mosby.

NANDA. (2001). *NANDA nursing diagnoses: Definitions & classification 2001–2002.* Philadelphia: Author.

Pender, N.J., Murdaugh, C.L. & Parsons, M.A. (2006). *Health promotion in nursing practice* (5th ed.). Upper Saddle River, NJ: Pearson Prentice-Hall.

Roget's II: The new thesaurus. (1980). Boston: Houghton Mifflin.

Figure 2.1 Taxonomy II Domains and Classes

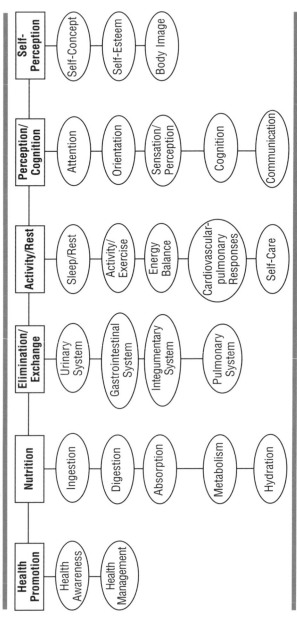
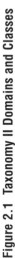

Figure 2.1 *continued*

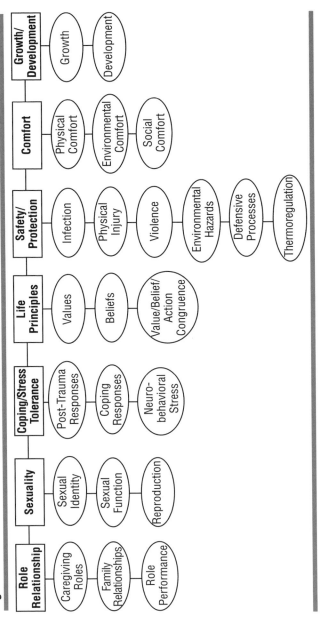

Figure 2.2 The ISO Reference Terminology Model for a Nursing Diagnosis

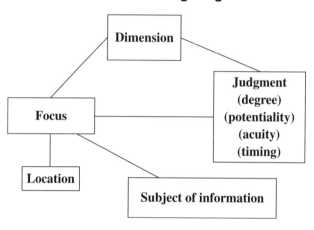

Figure 2.3 The NANDA-I Model of a Nursing Diagnosis

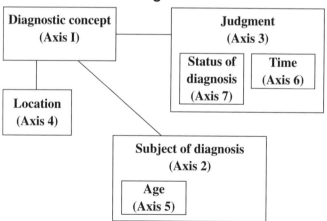

Figure 2.4 A NANDA-I Nursing Diagnosis
Model: *Ineffective Coping*

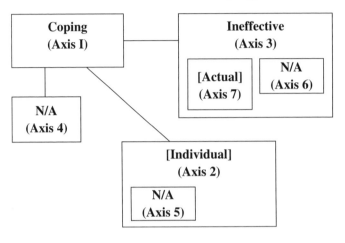

Figure 2.5 A NANDA-I Nursing Diagnosis
Model: *Risk for Impaired Parenting—*
Adolescent

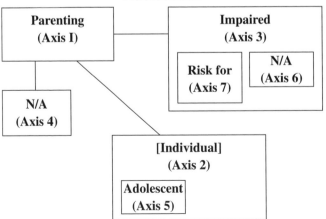

Figure 2.6 A NANDA-I Nursing Diagnosis Model: *Enhanced Coping—Family*

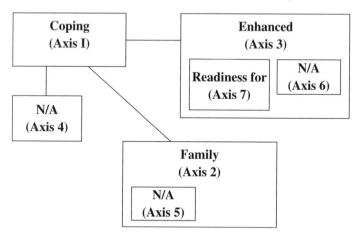

Table 2.1 Taxonomy II Domains, Classes, and Diagnoses

Domain 1 Health Promotion
The awareness of well-being or normality of function and the strategies used to maintain control of and enhance that well-being or normality of function

Class 1 Health Awareness Recognition of normal function and well-being

Class 2 Health Management Identifying, controlling, performing, and integrating activities to maintain health and well-being

Approved Diagnoses
00082	*Effective therapeutic regimen management*
00078	*Ineffective therapeutic regimen management*
00080	*Ineffective family therapeutic regimen management*
00081	*Ineffective community therapeutic regimen management*
00084	*Health-seeking behaviors (specify)*
00099	*Ineffective health maintenance*
00098	*Impaired home maintenance*
00162	*Readiness for enhanced therapeutic regimen management*
00163	*Readiness for enhanced nutrition*
00186	*Readiness for enhanced immunization status*

Domain 2 Nutrition
The activities of taking in, assimilating, and using nutrients for the purposes of tissue maintenance, tissue repair, and the production of energy

Class 1 Ingestion Taking food or nutrients into the body

Approved Diagnoses
00107	*Ineffective infant feeding pattern*
00103	*Impaired swallowing*
00002	*Imbalanced nutrition: Less than body requirements*
00001	*Imbalanced nutrition: More than body requirements*
00003	*Risk for imbalanced nutrition: More than body requirements*

Class 2 Digestion The physical and chemical activities that convert foodstuffs into substances suitable for absorption and assimilation

Class 3 Absorption The act of taking up nutrients through body tissues

continued

Table 2.1 *continued*

Class 4 Metabolism The chemical and physical processes occurring in living organisms and cells for the development and use of protoplasm, production of waste and energy, with the release of energy for all vital processes

Approved Diagnoses
00178	Risk for impaired liver function
00179	Risk for unstable blood glucose level

Class 5 Hydration The taking in and absorption of fluids and electrolytes

Approved Diagnoses
00027	Deficient fluid volume
00028	Risk for deficient fluid volume
00026	Excess fluid volume
00025	Risk for imbalanced fluid volume
00160	Readiness for enhanced fluid balance

Domain 3 Elimination and Exchange
Secretion and excretion of waste products from the body

Class 1 Urinary Function The process of secretion, reabsorption, and excretion of urine

Approved Diagnoses
00016	Impaired urinary elimination
00023	Urinary retention
00021	Total urinary incontinence
00020	Functional urinary incontinence
00017	Stress urinary incontinence
00019	Urge urinary incontinence
00018	Reflex urinary incontinence
00022	Risk for urge urinary incontinence
00166	Readiness for enhanced urinary elimination
00176	Overflow urinary incontinence

Class 2 Gastrointestinal Function The process of absorption and e cretion of the end products of digestion

Approved Diagnoses
00014	Bowel incontinence

00013   Diarrhea
00011   Constipation
00015   Risk for constipation
00012   Perceived constipation

Class 3 Integumentary Function The process of secretion and excretion through the skin

Class 4 Respiratory Function The process of exchange of gases and removal of the end products of metabolism

Approved Diagnoses
00030   Impaired gas exchange

Domain 4 Activity/Rest
The production, conservation, expenditure, or balance of energy resources

Class 1 Sleep/Rest Slumber, repose, ease, relaxation, or inactivity

Approved Diagnoses
00096   Sleep deprivation
00165   Readiness for enhanced sleep
00095   Insomnia

Class 2 Activity/Exercise Moving parts of the body (mobility), doing work, or performing actions often (but not always) against resistance

Approved Diagnoses
00040   Risk for disuse syndrome
00085   Impaired physical mobility
00091   Impaired bed mobility
00089   Impaired wheelchair mobility
00090   Impaired transfer ability
00088   Impaired walking
00097   Deficient diversional activity
00100   Delayed surgical recovery
00168   Sedentary lifestyle

continued

Table 2.1 *continued*

Class 3 Energy Balance A dynamic state of harmony between intake and expenditure of resources

Approved Diagnoses
00050   *Energy field disturbance*
00093   *Fatigue*

Class 4 Cardiovascular/Pulmonary Responses Cardiopulmonary mechanisms that support activity/rest

Approved Diagnoses
00029   *Decreased cardiac output*
00033   *Impaired spontaneous ventilation*
00032   *Ineffective breathing pattern*
00092   *Activity intolerance*
00094   *Risk for activity intolerance*
00034   *Dysfunctional ventilatory weaning response*
00024   *Ineffective tissue perfusion (specify type: renal, cerebral, cardiopulmonary, gastrointestinal, peripheral)*

Class 5. Self-Care Ability to perform activities to care for one's body and bodily functions

Approved Diagnoses
00109   *Dressing/grooming self-care deficit*
00108   *Bathing/hygiene self-care deficit*
00102   *Feeding self-care deficit*
00110   *Toileting self-care deficit*
00182   *Readiness for enhanced self-care*

Domain 5 Perception/Cognition
The human information processing system including attention, orientation, sensation, perception, cognition, and communication

Class 1 Attention Mental readiness to notice or observe

Approved Diagnoses
00123   *Unilateral neglect*

Class 2 Orientation Awareness of time, place, and person

Approved Diagnoses

00127   *Impaired environmental interpretation syndrome*
00154   *Wandering*

Class 3 Sensation/Perception Receiving information through the senses of touch, taste, smell, vision, hearing, and kinesthesia and the comprehension of sense data resulting in naming, associating, and/or pattern recognition

Approved Diagnoses

00122   *Disturbed sensory perception (specify: visual, auditory, kinesthetic, gustatory, tactile)*

Class 4 Cognition Use of memory, learning, thinking, problem solving, abstraction, judgment, insight, intellectual capacity, calculation, and language

Approved Diagnoses

00126   *Deficient knowledge (specify)*
00161   *Readiness for enhanced knowledge (specify)*
00128   *Acute confusion*
00129   *Chronic confusion*
00131   *Impaired memory*
00130   *Disturbed thought processes*
00184   *Readiness for enhanced decision making*
00173   *Risk for acute confusion*

Class 5 Communication Sending and receiving verbal and nonverbal information

Approved Diagnoses

00051   *Impaired verbal communication*
00157   *Readiness for enhanced communication*

Domain 6 Self-Perception

Awareness about the self

Class 1 Self-Concept The perception(s) about the total self

Approved Diagnoses

00121   *Disturbed personal identity*
00125   *Powerlessness*
00152   *Risk for powerlessness*
00124   *Hopelessness*

continued

Table 2.1 *continued*

00054	Risk for loneliness
00167	Readiness for enhanced self-concept
00187	Readiness for enhanced power
00174	Risk for compromised human dignity
00185	Readiness for enhanced hope

Class 2   Self-Esteem Assessment of one's own worth, capability, signifi-cance, and success

Approved Diagnoses

00119	Chronic low self-esteem
00120	Situational low self-esteem
00153	Risk for situational low self-esteem

Class 3   Body Image A mental image of one's own body

Approved Diagnoses

00118	Disturbed body image

Domain 7 Role Relationships

The positive and negative connections or associations between people or groups of people and the means by which those connections are demonstrated

Class 1   Caregiving Roles Socially expected behavior patterns by people providing care who are not healthcare professionals

Approved Diagnoses

00061	Caregiver role strain
00062	Risk for caregiver role strain
00056	Impaired parenting
00057	Risk for impaired parenting
00164	Readiness for enhanced parenting

Class 2   Family Relationships Associations of people who are biologically related or related by choice

Approved Diagnoses

00060	Interrupted family processes
00159	Readiness for enhanced family processes
00063	Dysfunctional family processes: Alcoholism
00058	Risk for impaired parent/infant/child attachment

Class 3 Role Performance Quality of functioning in socially expected behavior patterns

Approved Diagnoses
00106	*Effective breastfeeding*
00104	*Ineffective breastfeeding*
00105	*Interrupted breastfeeding*
00055	*Ineffective role performance*
00064	*Parental role conflict*
00052	*Impaired social interaction*

Domain 8 Sexuality
Sexual identity, sexual function, and reproduction

Class 1 Sexual Identity The state of being a specific person in regard to sexuality and/or gender

Class 2 Sexual Function The capacity or ability to participate in sexual activities

Approved Diagnoses
00059	*Sexual dysfunction*
00065	*Ineffective sexuality pattern*

Class 3 Reproduction Any process by which human beings are produced

Domain 9 Coping/Stress Tolerance
Contending with life events/life processes

Class 1 Post-Trauma Responses Reactions occurring after physical or psychological trauma

Approved Diagnoses
00114	*Relocation stress syndrome*
00149	*Risk for relocation stress syndrome*
00142	*Rape-trauma syndrome*
00144	*Rape-trauma syndrome: Silent reaction*
00143	*Rape-trauma syndrome: Compound reaction*
00141	*Post-trauma syndrome*
00145	*Risk for post-trauma syndrome*

Class 2 Coping Responses The process of managing environmental stress

continued

Table 2.1 *continued*

Approved Diagnoses

00148	*Fear*
00146	*Anxiety*
00147	*Death anxiety*
00137	*Chronic sorrow*
00072	*Ineffective denial*
00136	*Grieving*
00135	*Complicated grieving*
00069	*Ineffective coping*
00073	*Disabled family coping*
00074	*Compromised family coping*
00071	*Defensive coping*
00077	*Ineffective community coping*
00158	*Readiness for enhanced coping (individual)*
00075	*Readiness for enhanced family coping*
00076	*Readiness for enhanced community coping*
00172	*Risk for complicated grieving*
00177	*Stress overload*
00188	*Risk-prone health behavior*

Class 3 Neurobehavioral Stress Behavioral responses reflecting nerve and brain function

Approved Diagnoses

00009	*Autonomic dysreflexia*
00010	*Risk for autonomic dysreflexia*
00116	*Disorganized infant behavior*
00115	*Risk for disorganized infant behavior*
00117	*Readiness for enhanced organized infant behavior*
00049	*Decreased intracranial adaptive capacity*

Domain 10 Life Principles

Principles underlying conduct, thought, and behavior about acts, customs, or institutions viewed as being true or having intrinsic worth

Class 1 Values The identification and ranking of preferred modes of conduct or end states

Approved Diagnoses
00185   Readiness for enhanced hope

Class 2 Beliefs Opinions, expectations, or judgments about acts, customs, or institutions viewed as being true or having intrinsic worth

Approved Diagnoses
00068   Readiness for enhanced spiritual well-being
00185   Readiness for enhanced hope

Class 3 Value/Belief/Action Congruence The correspondence or balance achieved between values, beliefs, and actions

Approved Diagnoses
00066   Spiritual distress
00067   Risk for spiritual distress
00083   Decisional conflict (specify)
00079   Noncompliance (specify)
00170   Risk for impaired religiosity
00169   Impaired religiosity
00171   Readiness for enhanced religiosity
00175   Moral distress
00184   Readiness for enhanced decision making

Domain 11 Safety/Protection
Freedom from danger, physical injury, or immune system damage; preservation from loss; and protection of safety and security

Class 1 Infection Host responses following pathogenic invasion

Approved Diagnoses
00004   Risk for infection
00186   Readiness for enhanced immunization status

Class 2 Physical Injury Bodily harm or hurt

Approved Diagnoses
00045   Impaired oral mucous membrane
00035   Risk for injury
00087   Risk for perioperative positioning injury
00155   Risk for falls
00038   Risk for trauma

continued

Table 2.1 *continued*

00046	*Impaired skin integrity*
00047	*Risk for impaired skin integrity*
00044	*Impaired tissue integrity*
00048	*Impaired dentition*
00036	*Risk for suffocation*
00039	*Risk for aspiration*
00031	*Ineffective airway clearance*
00086	*Risk for peripheral neurovascular dysfunction*
00043	*Ineffective protection*
00156	*Risk for sudden infant death syndrome*

Class 3 Violence The exertion of excessive force or power so as to cause injury or abuse

Approved Diagnoses
00139	*Risk for self-mutilation*
00151	*Self-mutilation*
00138	*Risk for other-directed violence*
00140	*Risk for self-directed violence*
00150	*Risk for suicide*

Class 4 Environmental Hazards Sources of danger in the surroundings

Approved Diagnoses
00037	*Risk for poisoning*
00180	*Risk for contamination*
00181	*Contamination*

Class 5 Defensive Processes The processes by which the self protects itself from the nonself

Approved Diagnoses
00041	*Latex allergy response*
00042	*Risk for latex allergy response*
00186	*Readiness for enhanced immunization status*

Class 6 Thermoregulation The physiologic process of regulating heat and energy within the body for purposes of protecting the organism

Approved Diagnoses
00005	*Risk for imbalanced body temperature*

00008	Ineffective thermoregulation
00006	Hypothermia
00007	Hyperthermia

Domain 12 Comfort
Sense of mental, physical, or social well-being or ease

Class 1 Physical Comfort Sense of well-being or ease and/or freedom from pain

Approved Diagnoses
00132	Acute pain
00133	Chronic pain
00134	Nausea
00183	Readiness for enhanced comfort

Class 2 Environmental Comfort Sense of well-being or ease in/with one's environment

Approved Diagnoses
00183	Readiness for enhanced comfort

Class 3 Social Comfort Sense of well-being or ease with one's social situations

Approved Diagnoses
00053	Social isolation

Domain 13 Growth/Development
Age-appropriate increases in physical dimensions, maturation of organ systems, and/or progression through the developmental milestone

Class 1 Growth Increases in physical dimensions or maturity of organ systems

Approved Diagnoses
00111	Delayed growth and development
00113	Risk for disproportionate growth
00101	Adult failure to thrive

Class 2 Development Progression or regression through a sequence of recognized milestones in life

Approved Diagnoses
00111	Delayed growth and development
00112	Risk for delayed development

Table 2.2 NNN Taxonomy of Nursing Practice: Placement of Nursing Diagnoses

Domains	*Classes*	*Diagnoses, Outcomes, and Interventions*	*NANDA-I Nursing Diagnoses*
I. Functional Includes diagnoses, outcomes, and interventions to promote basic needs	**Activity/Exercise**	Physical activity, including energy conservation and expenditure	*Activity intolerance* *Risk for activity intolerance* *Risk for disuse syndrome* *Risk for falls* *Fatigue* *Impaired bed mobility* *Impaired physical mobility* *Impaired wheelchair mobility* *Impaired transfer ability* *Impaired walking* *Sedentary lifestyle*
	Comfort	A sense of emotional, physical, and spiritual well being and relative freedom from distress	*Nausea* *Acute pain* *Chronic pain* *Disturbed energy field* *Readiness for enhanced comfort*
	Growth and Development	Physical, emotional, and social growth and development milestones	*Risk for delayed development* *Adult failure to thrive*

		Delayed growth and development *Risk for disproportionate growth* *Disorganized infant behavior* *Risk for disorganized infant behavior* *Readiness for enhanced organized infant behavior*
Nutrition	Processes related to taking in, assimilating, and using nutrients	*Effective breastfeeding* *Ineffective breastfeeding* *Interrupted breastfeeding* *Ineffective infant feeding pattern* *Imbalanced nutrition: Less than body requirements* *Imbalanced nutrition: More than body requirements* *Risk for imbalanced nutrition: More than body requirements* *Readiness for enhanced nutrition* *Impaired swallowing*
Self-Care	Ability to accomplish basic and instrumental activities of daily living	*Bathing/hygiene self-care deficit* *Dressing/grooming self-care deficit* *Feeding self-care deficit* *Toileting self-care deficit* *Readiness for enhanced self-care*

continued

Table 2.2 *continued*

Domains	Classes	Diagnoses, Outcomes, and Interventions	NANDA-I Nursing Diagnoses
I. Functional (*continued*)	**Sexuality**	Maintenance or modification of sexual identity and patterns	*Sexual dysfunction* *Ineffective sexuality patterns*
	Sleep/Rest	The quantity and quality of sleep, rest and relaxation patterns	*Sleep deprivation* *Insomnia* *Readiness for enhanced sleep*
	Values/Beliefs	Ideas, goals, perceptions, spiritual and other beliefs that influence choices or decisions	*Spiritual distress* *Risk for spiritual distress* *Readiness for enhanced spiritual well-being* *Impaired religiosity* *Risk for impaired religiosity* *Readiness for enhanced religiosity* *Moral distress*

II. Physiological
Includes diagnoses, outcomes, and interventions to promote optimal biophysical health

Cardiac Function	Cardiac mechanisms used to maintain tissue profusion	*Decreased cardiac output*
		Ineffective tissue perfusion
Elimination	Processes related to secretion and excretion of body wastes	*Bowel incontinence*
		Constipation
		Perceived constipation
		Risk for constipation
		Diarrhea
		Functional urinary incontinence
		Reflex urinary incontinence
		Stress urinary incontinence
		Total urinary incontinence
		Urge urinary incontinence
		Risk for urge urinary incontinence
		Impaired urinary elimination
		Urinary retention
		Readiness for enhanced urinary elimination
		Overflow incontinence
Fluid & Electrolyte	Regulation of fluids/electrolytes and acid base balance	*Deficient fluid volume*
		Excess fluid volume
		Risk for deficient fluid volume

continued

Table 2.2 *continued*

Domains	Classes	Diagnoses, Outcomes, and Interventions	NANDA-I Nursing Diagnoses
II. Physiological *(continued)*			Risk for imbalanced fluid volume Readiness for enhanced fluid balance
	Neurocognition	Mechanisms related to the nervous system and neurocognitive functioning, including memory, thinking, and judgment	Autonomic dysreflexia Risk for autonomic dysreflexia Acute confusion Chronic confusion Risk for acute confusion Impaired environmental interpretation syndrome Decreased intracranial adaptive capacity Impaired memory Unilateral neglect Disturbed thought processes Wandering

Pharmacological Function	Effects (therapeutic and adverse) of medications or drugs and other pharmacologically active products	
Physical Regulation	Body temperature, endocrine, and immune system responses to regulate cellular processes	*Latex allergy response* *Risk for latex allergy response* *Risk for imbalanced body temperature* *Hyperthermia* *Hypothermia* *Ineffective thermoregulation* *Risk for infection* *Risk for peripheral neurovascular dysfunction* *Ineffective protection* *Risk for unstable blood sugar* *Risk for impaired liver function*
Reproduction	Processes related to human procreation and birth	
Respiratory Function	Ventilation adequate to maintain arterial blood gases within normal limits	*Ineffective airway clearance* *Risk for aspiration*

continued

Table 2.2 *continued*

Domains	Classes	Diagnoses, Outcomes, and Interventions	NANDA-I Nursing Diagnoses
II. Psychosocial *(continued)*			Ineffective breathing pattern Impaired gas exchange Risk for suffocation Impaired spontaneous ventilation Dysfunctional ventilatory weaning response
	Sensation/Perception	Intake and interpretation of information through the senses, including seeing, hearing, touching, tasting, smelling	Disturbed sensory perception
	Tissue Integrity	Skin and mucous membrane protection to support secretion, excretion, and healing	Impaired dentition Impaired oral mucous membrane Impaired skin integrity Risk for impaired skin integrity Impaired tissue integrity

III. Psychosocial
Includes diagnoses, outcomes, and interventions to promote optimal mental and emotional health and social functioning

Behavior
Actions that promote, maintain, or restore health

Ineffective health maintenance
Health-seeking behaviors
Noncompliance
Effective therapeutic regimen management
Ineffective therapeutic regimen management
Ineffective community therapeutic regimen management
Ineffective family therapeutic regimen management
Readiness for enhanced therapeutic regimen management

Communication
Receiving, interpreting, and expressing spoken, written, and nonverbal messages

Impaired verbal communication
Readiness for enhanced communication

Coping
Adjusting or adapting to stressful events

Risk-prone health behavior
Decisional conflict
Ineffective coping
Ineffective community coping

continued

Table 2.2 *continued*

Domains	Classes	Diagnoses, Outcomes, and Interventions	NANDA-I Nursing Diagnoses
III. **Psychosocial** (*continued*)			Readiness for enhanced community coping
			Defensive coping
			Compromised family coping
			Disabled family coping
			Readiness for enhanced family coping
			Ineffective denial
			Grieving
			Complicated grieving
			Risk for complicated grieving
			Post-trauma syndrome
			Risk for post-trauma syndrome
			Rape-trauma syndrome
			Rape-trauma syndrome: Compound reaction
			Rape-trauma syndrome: Silent reaction
			Relocation stress syndrome
			Risk for relocation stress syndrome

		Self-mutilation
		Risk for self-mutilation
		Risk for suicide
		Risk for self-directed violence
		Readiness for enhanced coping
		Stress overload
		Readiness for enhanced decision making
Emotional	A mental state or feeling that may influence perceptions of the world	Anxiety
		Death anxiety
		Fear
		Hopelessness
		Chronic sorrow
		Readiness for enhanced hope
Knowledge	Understanding and skill in applying information to promote, maintain, and restore health	Deficient knowledge (specify)
		Readiness for enhanced knowledge (specify)
Roles/Relationships	Maintenance and/or modification of expected social behaviors and emotional connectedness with others	Risk for impaired parent/child attachment
		Caregiver role strain

continued

Table 2.2 *continued*

Domains	Classes	Diagnoses, Outcomes, and Interventions	NANDA-I Nursing Diagnoses
III. **Psychosocial** *(continued)*			*Risk for caregiver role strain*
			Parental role conflict
			Dysfunctional family processes: alcoholism
			Interrupted family processes
			Impaired parenting
			Risk for impaired parenting
			Ineffective role performance
			Impaired social interaction
			Social isolation
			Risk for other-directed violence
			Readiness for enhanced family processes
			Readiness for enhanced parenting
	Self-Perception	Awareness of one's body and personal identity	*Disturbed body image*
			Disturbed personal identity
			Risk for loneliness
			Powerlessness

Risk for powerlessness
Chronic low self-esteem
Situational low self-esteem
Risk for situational low self-esteem
Readiness for enhanced self-concept
Readiness for enhanced power
Risk for compromised human dignity

IV. Environmental
Includes diagnoses, outcomes, and interventions to promote and protect the environmental health and safety of individuals, systems, and communities

Healthcare System
Social, political, and economic structures and processes for the delivery of health-care services

Populations
Aggregates of individuals or communities having characteristics in common

Risk Management
Avoidance of identifiable health threats

Impaired home maintenance
Risk for injury
Risk for perioperative positioning injury
Risk for poisoning
Risk for trauma

continued

Table 2.2 *continued*

Domains	Classes	Diagnoses, Outcomes, and Interventions	NANDA-I Nursing Diagnoses
IV. Environmental *(continued)*			*Risk for sudden infant death syndrome*
			Readiness for enhanced immunization
			Contamination
			Risk for contamination

Unable to place in the structure:
Deficient diversional activity
Delayed surgical recovery

This structure is in the public domain and can be freely used without permission; neither the structure nor a modification can be copyrighted by any person, group, or organization; any use of the structure should acknowledge the source.

Part 3

NURSING DIAGNOSIS: APPLICATIONS AND SUBMISSION GUIDELINES

2007–2008

Nursing Diagnosis in Education

Martha Craft-Rosenberg, PhD, RN, FAAN,
and Kelly Smith, MSN, RN

The use of nursing diagnoses is central to nursing education. The assessment and diagnosis of individuals, families,
and communities teaches students hypothetical reasoning
and critical thinking. Further, those who come to nurses for
assistance expect the achievement of improved health outcomes for which nurses are increasingly held accountable.
Outcomes and the selection of interventions rest on accurate
and valid nursing diagnoses.

Teaching nursing students to use nursing diagnoses begins
with assessment and history-taking. As students assess and
collect data (information) regarding individuals, families, and
communities, they are identifying the "signs and symptoms"
or defining characteristics of the nursing diagnoses concepts.
The factors or variables influencing diagnoses are integrated
with the history, charts, and other evidence. These variables
provide the context, the "related factors," that are combined
with the defining characteristics to make nursing diagnoses.
When possible, nurses treat related factors with interventions
to prevent or reduce their impact. When it is not possible for
nurses to treat a related factor, they treat the defining characteristics with selected nursing interventions.

The book you are reading includes the complete list of
nursing diagnoses terms (concepts), defining characteristics,
related factors, and risk factors. This book is published
every two years by NANDA International. It is small enough
for nursing students to carry a copy with them on clinical
units in acute care and community settings. Anyone can
purchase copies from NANDA International's Web site
(www.nanda.org).

Assessment and Identifying Defining Characteristics

The defining characteristics are those characteristics in individuals, families, and communities that are observable and

verifiable. They serve as cues or inferences that cluster as manifestations of an actual illness or wellness health state, or nursing diagnosis. Suppose, for example, an individual (Sarah) states to a nursing student that she is "sick to my stomach" and asks for an emesis basin. The nursing student further observes that Sarah is swallowing a great deal and gagging. These defining characteristics are suggestive of the nursing diagnosis *nausea.*

History and Identifying Related Factors

The related factors provide the context for the defining characteristics. Related factors are factors that appear to show some type of patterned relationship with the nursing diagnosis. These factors may be described as antecedent to, associated with, related to, contributing to, or abetting the diagnosis. They are identified as characteristics or history of individuals, families, and communities. In the case of Sarah, she may tell us that she is taking large doses of aspirin on the advice of her physician, and that she takes the aspirin on an empty stomach. In this case students can establish an "outcome of freedom from nausea" and use the NIC nursing intervention of "Nausea Management" (Dochterman & Bulechek, 2004), especially the activity of "Reduce or eliminate personal factors that precipitate or increase the nausea (taking aspirin on an empty stomach)."

Selecting the Nursing Diagnosis Label

The nursing diagnosis label is selected based upon two characteristics. First, the definition of the diagnosis label should convey a combination of the defining characteristics and related factors. Second, the diagnosis selected is the term with defining characteristics and related factors that fit the data students collect on assessment and history taking. In this case the definition of *nausea* is "A subjective unpleasant, wavelike sensation in the back of the throat, epigastrium, or abdomen that may lead to the urge or need to vomit" (p. 142). In the example, Sarah stated that she is "sick to my stomach" and exhibited other defining characteristics. Her history provided an antecedent of nausea—the ingestion of large doses of aspirin on an empty stomach.

Risk Diagnoses

Nurses have always been responsible to identify individuals, families, and communities at risk and protect them from this risk. A risk diagnoses "describes human responses to health conditions/life processes that may develop in a vulnerable individual, family, or community. It is supported by risk factors that contribute to increased vulnerability" (p. 332). For example, the diagnosis of *risk for impaired skin integrity* includes both internal and external factors that influence vulnerability. The interventions a nurse selects to reach the outcomes are based on these influencing factors.

Health-Promotion Diagnoses

A health-promotion diagnosis is a clinical judgment of a person's, family's, or community's motivation and desire to increase well-being and actualize human health potential as expressed in their readiness to enhance specific health behaviors such as nutrition and exercise. Health-promotion diagnoses can be used in any health state and do not require current levels of wellness. This readiness is supported by defining characteristics. Interventions are selected in concert with the individual/family/community to best ensure the ability to reach the stated outcomes.

Wellness Diagnoses

A wellness diagnosis describes human responses to levels of wellness in an individual, family, or community that have a readiness for enhancement. This readiness is supported by defining characteristics. As with all diagnoses, nurse-sensitive (sensitive to nursing interventions) outcomes are identified and nursing interventions are selected that provide a high likelihood of reaching the outcomes.

Prioritizing Diagnoses

Prioritizing diagnoses is one type of critical thinking that most nursing educators expect from students. Faculty members often request a list of nursing diagnoses from students. Students compile this list while they are reading the history of individuals, families, and communities. After assessment, the students need to make decisions regarding prioritizing diagnoses. Priorities are established based upon the needs of individuals, families, and communities. When nursing students are assigned to clinical experience for a short period of time, faculty members may ask them to choose nursing diagnoses they can address during this time frame.

Linking Nursing Diagnoses to Outcomes and Interventions

Accurate and valid nursing diagnoses determine the nurse-sensitive outcomes. These outcomes guide the selection of interventions that are likely to produce the desired treatment effects. Again, interventions will treat either related factors (or risk factors) or defining characteristics. Faculty members and their students can use the linkage book (Johnson et al., 2006) or the linkages to nursing diagnoses provided in the back of the NIC (Dochterman & Bulechek, 2004) and NOC (Moorhead, Johnson, & Maas, 2004) books. These linkages with nursing diagnoses provide clear examples for linking diagnoses, interventions, and outcomes. Some faculty members, however, may require their students to identify outcomes and select nursing interventions independently in order to apply critical thinking skills.

Faculty members using nursing diagnoses will detect an increase in critical and analytical thinking from students, which will have a clear focus on prioritized individual, family, and community needs. Faculty members who are new to this process will learn with their students initially, but both will be amazed at the speed with which this "natural" process is applied.

References

Dochterman, J.M., & Bulechek, G. (Eds.). (2004). *Nursing interventions classification* (NIC). St. Louis, MO: Mosby.

Johnson, J., Bulechek, G., Butcher, H., Dochterman, J., Maas, M., Moorhead, S., & Swanson, E. (2006). *NANDA, NOC, and NIC Linkages: Nursing diagnoses, outcomes, & interventions* (2nd ed.). St. Louis, MO: Mosby.

Moorhead, S., Johnson, M., & Maas, M. (Eds.). (2004*). Nursing outcomes classification* (NOC). St. Louis, MO..

The Value of Nursing Diagnoses in Electronic Health Records

Jane Brokel, PhD, RN, and Crystal Heath, MSN, RN

In 2004, the healthcare industry accounted for $1.9 trillion dollars, 16% of the United States Gross Domestic Product (Doeksen, 2006). MECON (1995) and the Healthcare Financial Management Association in 1995 reported that nursing labor costs accounted for more than 50% of the total healthcare labor costs. As a result, in the mid-1990s hospital corporations reduced labor costs by reducing nursing personnel (DeMoro, 2000; Wunderlich, Sloan, & Davis, 1996). Consequently, the prospective payment system was driving the reductions in inpatient admissions and lengths of stay while hospitals experienced increasing complexity of care for inpatients. Additionally, the prospective payment system was moving care from the hospital settings to other ambulatory settings such as home care. These changes have implications for nursing labor resource requirements (Kovner, Jones, & Gergen, 2000). Yet no specific nursing data was ever used to guide the decisions on where reduction of personnel should occur.

Previous studies had found that nursing diagnoses associated with each patient explained a portion of length of hospital stay, ICU length of stay, and total hospital charges (Welton & Halloran, 1999). Nursing diagnoses also explained a portion of the number of home health nursing visits (Marek, 1996). Titler and team (2006) studied the movement of patients with hip fractures from the hospital. Her team found the documented nursing interventions provided during hospital care predicted whether the patients were discharged home or to another intermediate nursing facility setting. In view of the fact that nursing interventions and costs are a significant source of hospital expenditures, there is still very little quantitative analysis on nurses' contributions to overall patient outcomes. Now, nurse-staffing levels are under continual review with even legislative debates to determine ratios of nurses to patients. Using standardized nursing languages within clinical information systems can provide nurses and others with the information that demonstrates contributions of nursing care (Titler et al., 2006). These complex studies compile the data from multiple healthcare information systems and even paper systems, which have a wide variation in documentation methods.

Nursing services are not always identified as revenue-generating for a hospital since nursing services historically have been included as overhead in the room and board (Hendricks & Baume, 1997). Since the care provided by nurses has not been collected and analyzed, the effect on outcomes and the benefits of nursing assessments, interventions, and coordination of care for the patient and hospital are not quantified. In order to provide the quantifiable information required to effectively evaluate the value of nursing, standardized nursing terminologies must be uniformly included in the electronic health record (EHR) so the data are systematically collected and analyzed (Lavin, Avant, Craft-Rosenberg, Herdman, & Gebbie, 2004).

Since nursing personnel are the main source of hospital expenditures, the ability to extract standard nursing terms from the EHR will provide answers for the management of healthcare costs. Nursing data are more important than ever in today's environment in order to improve patient safety and manage health care efficiently and cost effectively (Jerant, Azairn, & Nesbitt, 2001). Cost-effectiveness analysis is dependent on an ingredients method (Levin & McEwan, 2001). Basically, every intervention uses ingredients that have a value or costs. If the ingredients can be *identified* and their costs ascertained, then the total cost of the intervention and the cost per unit of effectiveness, benefit, or utility can be calculated (Levin & McEwan). Terminologies such as NANDA nursing diagnoses, NIC interventions, NOC outcomes and indicators, when used in conjunction with each other, provide the best opportunity to answer questions about the safety, efficiency, and cost-effectiveness of nursing practice for patient populations. Several frameworks have been proposed to use the terminologies together in EHRs, such as VIPS Models (Ehnforss, Ehrenberg, & Thorell-Ekstand, 1998), OPT Model (Pesut & Herman, 1999), NNN Taxonomy of Nursing Practice (Mc-

Closkey, & Bulechek, 2004), and the KPO Model (von Krogh, Dale, & Naden, 2005)

Nursing documentation in current practice primarily consists of lengthy, paper-based, narrative notes. This approach has significant variations in terms to describe nursing findings and actions, and therefore disadvantages anyone's ability to analyze care. Narrative notes are ambiguous, contain redundancies and various nuances within the text. In addition, since these notes are usually handwritten, they are frequently illegible, misinterpreted, and are generally available only to one person at a time. As a result of these issues, narrative notes are difficult to enter into a computerized system where they can be retrieved for daily evaluation of patient care or analyzed for research and decision support (Bates, Ebell, Gotlieb, Zapp, & Mullins, 2003).

The inclusion of nursing diagnoses in conjunction with the Nursing Intervention Classification (McCloskey & Bulechek, 2004) and the Nursing Outcome Classification (Moorhead, Johnson, & Maas, 2004) in the EHR provides a comprehensive means for capturing the unique contribution of nursing in a consistent and quantifiable format. This consistency can provide the following benefits:

- Facilitate communication efforts of the healthcare team. These nursing terms along with uniform medication and medical terms will provide continuity of care within nursing units and across nursing settings (Figoski & Downey, 2006).
- A language that links nursing concepts for the nursing process within the EHR and facilitates the eventual data exchange of nursing process concepts.
- A means of describing the knowledge and skills essential to nursing practice (Lunney, 2006).
- A common method to allow nurse executives and administrators to collect and analyze nursing-specific data that will provide evidence of the effects and contributions nursing care provides, as well as the ability to cost out nursing services to third party payers (Jerant et al., 2001).

- A common means to capture data on patient outcomes that will assist design and build new knowledge to support evidence-based practice (Lavin et al., 2004).
- A mechanism to facilitate health ministry and legislative debate with policy development (Lavin et al., 2004).
- A common language in the education process to teach clinical decision making to nursing students (Garcia, Hansche, & Lobert, 2006; Gloskey, Kravutske, & Zugcic, 2006; Gordon, 2006; Johnson, 2006).
- Information to advance the science of nursing care.
- In order for the EHR to truly reflect the total care provided by healthcare professionals, it must include nursing data to reflect the nursing process (von Krogh et al., 2005).

Standardized nursing terminologies such as NANDA, NIC, and NOC provide the means of collecting nursing data that are systematically analyzed within and across healthcare organizations. Furthermore, these data are essential to provide the foundation for any cost/benefit analysis for nursing practice.

References

Bates, D.W., Ebell, M., Gotlieb, E., Zapp, J., & Mullins, H.C. (2003). A proposal for electronic medical records in U.S. primary care. *Journal of the American Medical Informatics Association, 10*(1), 1–10.

DeMoro, D. (2000). Engineering a crisis. How hospitals created a shortage of nurses. *Revolution, 1*(2), 16–23.

Doeksen, G.A. (2006). *The changing face of economic development: Health care as an economic engine.* Paper presented at the EcoMod International Conference on Regional and Urban Modeling, Brussels, Belgium.

Ehnfors, M., Ehrenberg, A., & Thorell-Ekstand, I. (1998). *VIPS boken. The VIPS book.* Stockholm: Vordforbunder.

Figoski, M., & Downey, J. (2006). Perspectives in continuity of care. Facility charging and nursing intervention classification (NIC): The new dynamic duo. *Nursing Economics,* 24, 102–111.

Garcia, T., Hansche, J., & Lobert, J.H. (2006). A user's guide to operationalizing NANDA, NIC, and NOC in a nursing curriculum. *The International Journal of Nursing Terminologies & Classifications,* (17), 33–34.

Gloskey, D., Kravutske, M.E., & Zugcic, M. (2006). Do you need to educate RNs on how to document using the nursing outcome classification? *The International Journal of Nursing Terminologies & Classifications. (17)*, 34–35.

Gordon, M. (2006). Tips on teaching nursing diagnosis. *The International Journal of Nursing Terminologies & Classifications, (17)*, 35.

Hendricks, J., & Baume, P. (1997). The pricing of nursing care. *Journal of Advanced Nursing, 25*, 454–462.

Jerant, A.F., Azari, R., & Nesbitt, T.S. (2001). Reducing the cost of frequent hospital admissions for congestive heart failure. A randomized trial of a home telecare intervention. *Medical Care, 39*, 1234–1245.

Johnson, M. (2006). Linking NANDA, NOC and NIC. *The International Journal of Nursing Terminologies & Classifications, 17*, 39–40.

Kovner, C.T., Jones, C.B., & Gergen, P.J. (2000). Nursing staffing in acute care hospitals, 1990–1996. *Policy, Politics, & Nursing Practice, 1*, 194–204.

Lavin, M.A., Avant, K., Craft-Rosenberg, M., Herdman, T.H., & Gebbie, K. (2004). Contexts for the study of the economic influence of nursing diagnoses on patient outcomes. *International Journal of Nursing Terminologies and Classifications, 15*, 39–47.

Levin, H.M., & McEwan, P.J. (2001). *Cost-effectiness analysis* (2nd ed.). Thousand Oaks, CA: Sage.

Lunney, M. (2006). Staff development. Helping nurses use NANDA, NOC, and NIC: Novice to expert. *Journal of Nursing Administration, 36*, 118–125.

Marek, K.D. (1996). Nursing diagnoses and home care nursing utilization. *Public Health Nurse, 13*, 195–200.

McCloskey, J., & Bulechek, G. (2004). *Nursing interventions classification* (NIC, 4th ed.). St. Louis, MO: Mosby.

MECON and Healthcare Financial Management Association. (1995). *From increasing revenues to controlling costs: Benchmark data for strategic planning [Supplement]*. Westchester, IL: Author..

Moorhead, S., Johnson, M., & Maas, M. (2004). *Nursing outcomes classification* (NOC). St. Louis, MO: Mosby.

Pesut, D.J., & Herman, J. (1999). Clinical reasoning. *The art & science of critical & creative thinking*. Detroit, MI: Delmar.

Titler, M., Dochterman, J., Xie, X., Kanak, M., Fei, Q., Piconi, D.M., & Shever, L. (2006). Nursing interventions and other factors associated with discharge disposition in older patients after hip fractures. *Nursing Research, 55*, 231–242.

von Krogh, G., Dale, C., & Naden, D. (2005). A framework for integrating NANDA, NIC, and NOC terminology in electronic patient records. *Journal of Nursing Scholarship, 37,* 275–281.

Welton, J.M., & Halloran, E.J. (1999). A comparison of nursing and medical diagnoses in predicting hospital outcomes. Transforming health care through informatics: Cornerstone for a new information management paradigm. *Proceedings from AMIA 1999 Annual Symposium* (pp. 171–175). Bethesda, MD: AMIA.

Wunderlich, G., Sloan, F., & Davis, C. (Eds.). (1996). *Nursing staff in hospitals and nursing homes: Is it adequate?* Washington, DC: National Academy Press.

Nursing Diagnosis and Research

Margaret Lunney, PhD, RN

Since 1973, the diagnoses approved for the NANDA-I Taxonomy of Nursing Diagnoses were developed and submitted by nurses using a variety of research methods. Each diagnosis is research-based, with some diagnoses having stronger research evidence than others. Over the last four decades, the research methods have become more sophisticated and the Diagnosis Development Committee has required more stringent evidence as the basis for approving new diagnoses.

To remain evidence-based, however, the NANDA-I Taxonomy needs ongoing research support (Whitley, 1999). Some of the types of studies needed are concept analyses, content validation, construct and criterion-related validation, consensus validation, and studies of accuracy of nurses' diagnoses. The references cited can be used as resources for these research methods.

Concept Analyses

Concept development and analyses have been and continue to be an important aspect of development and approval of new diagnoses (Avant, 1990). Concept identification and formulation is the first step in developing a new diagnoses and refining previously accepted diagnoses. Each nursing diagnosis is a concept that needs to be developed using systematic methods (Walker & Avant, 2005). A classic study, for example, was Whitley's (1992) concept analysis of *fear*. At the 2006 NNN Alliance conference, a concept analysis was reported to develop a new wellness-health promotion diagnosis: *Supportive Family Role Performance* (Lamont, 2006).

Content Validation

Content validation studies are often foundational for refining approved diagnoses and developing new diagnoses. In these studies, there are two possible groups of subjects—

nurses who work with patients who experience the specific diagnoses or patients who currently are experiencing the diagnosis (Fehring, 1986). A problem with nurses as subjects, however, especially if it is a new diagnosis, is that they are being asked to state from memory the relevance of defining characteristics. Clinical validation studies, in which patients are assessed for defining characteristics at the time they experience the specific human response, provide better data for content validation studies.

For decades, the data from clinical validation studies have served as support for nursing diagnoses, e.g., Bartek, Lindeman, and Hawks (1999), Carlson-Catalano et al., (1998), and Kim et al. (1984). The challenges of conducting clinical studies are significant but worthwhile since data are from actual patients who are presently experiencing the human response of interest to the researcher. Methodological considerations for such studies were described by Carlson-Catalano and Lunney (1995); Grant, Kinney, and Guzzetta (1990); and Maas, Hardy, and Craft (1990). Sparks and Lien-Gieschen (1994) provided revised guidelines for scoring and interpreting defining characteristics as highly or moderately relevant for making a diagnosis. These scoring revisions are important to avoid development of long lists of defining characteristics. Some of the currently approved diagnoses have long lists of defining characteristics that could be reduced if clinical studies were done using the aforementioned guidelines.

Construct and Criterion-Related Validity

"Knowledge development of diagnoses in the NANDA taxonomy means a series of studies needs to be done for each individual diagnosis as well as groups of diagnoses" (Parker & Lunney, 1998, p. 146). The various types of studies needed to establish construct and criterion-related validity are reliability, epidemiological, outcome, causal analysis, and generalizability studies (Parker & Lunney). Reliability studies can establish the stability and coherence of diagnoses. Epidemiological studies of the incidence and prevalence of specific diagnoses in settings and populations can show the importance and co-occurrence of diagnoses. For example, in retrospective analyses of 123, 241 sequential admissions to a university hospital, Welton and Halloran (2005) demonstrated that nursing diagnoses were good predictors of hospital outcomes, adding 30% to 146% of explanatory power to diagnosis-related groups (DRGs) and all payer-refined DRGs. Epidemiological studies can also be done to show the relationship among diagnoses, interventions, and outcomes. Outcome, or effectiveness, studies can illustrate the prognoses of diagnoses and the best interventions to help people who are experiencing specific diagnoses. A symposia of three examples of effectiveness studies was presented at the 2006 NNN Alliance conference (Dochterman, 2006). Causal analysis studies, using experimental designs, can show the relation of diagnoses to theories and the importance of using standardized diagnoses to achieve high quality nursing care. Generalizability studies can show the importance of nursing diagnoses across institutions and medical diagnoses or ICD-9 categories. A good resource for conducting validity and reliability studies is a book on measurement (e.g., Waltz, Strickland, & Lenz, 2005).

Consensus Validation

Consensus validation techniques are being used to establish the connections of NANDA, NIC, and NOC with specific populations for purposes of developing standards of practice and identifying the specific terms to be included in electronic health records (Carlson, 2006a, 2006b; Minthorn, 2006; Westmoreland, Wesorick, Hanson, & Wyngarden, 2000). Westmoreland et al.'s study validated that their clinical practice guidelines delineated "the right services and knowledge related to these services" (p. 19). Carlson (2006a) recommends participatory action research methods for practicing nurses to identify the specific NANDA, NIC, and NOC terms that apply to patients served by their agency or unit. This process is being used in a variety of settings and can be adopted by nurses in any setting and locality. In the near future, the Research Committee will be promoting this process as a standardized method to establish standards of practice and to select terms for electronic health records.

Studies of Accuracy of Nurses' Diagnoses

Studies of accuracy of nurses' diagnoses and factors that influence accuracy are needed because previous studies established that accuracy varies widely (Lunney, 2001). The accuracy of nurses' diagnoses is important because this is the foundation for choices of interventions and outcomes. Accuracy studies are described in the Appendix of Lunney (2001) and were presented at the 2006 NNN Alliance Conference (Crossetti, & Saurin, 2006; Hasegawa et al., 2006).

Summary

Nursing diagnosis studies are sorely needed to maintain and enhance the evidence-base of the NANDA International Taxonomy. The Research Committee is eager to provide assistance to anyone considering undertaking a study. Contact margell@si.rr.com or Lunney@mail.csi.cuny.edu.

References

Avant, K.C. (1990). The art and science in nursing diagnosis development. *Nursing Diagnosis, 1*(2), 51–56.

Bartek, J.K., Lindeman, M., & Hawks, J.H. (1999). Clinical validation of characteristics of the alcoholic family. *Nursing Diagnosis: The Journal of Nursing Language and Classification, 10, 158–168.*

Carlson, J.M. (2006a). Consensus validation process: A standardized research method to identify and link their relevant NANDA, NIC and NOC terms for local populations [Abstract]. *International Journal of Nursing Terminologies and Classifications, 17* (1), 23–24.

Carlson, J.M. (2006b). Professional nursing latent tuberculosis infection standards of practice development using NANDA, NIC and NOC [Abstract]. *International Journal of Nursing Terminologies and Classifications, 17* (1), 62.

Carlson-Catalano, J., & Lunney, M. (1995). Quantitative methods for clinical validation of nursing diagnoses. *Clinical Nurse Specialist: The Journal of Advanced Nursing Practice, 9,* 306–311.

Carlson-Catalano, J., Lunney, M., Paradiso, C., Bruno, J., Luise, B.K., Martin, T., Massoni, M., & Pachter, S. (1998). Clinical validation of ineffective breathing pattern, ineffective airway clearance and impaired gas exchange. *IMAGE: Journal of Nursing Scholarship, 30,* 243–248.

Crossetti, M.G.O., & Saurin, G. (2006). Critical thinking and nursing diagnosis accuracy in a university hospital [Abstract]. *International Journal of Nursing Terminologies and Classifications, 17,* 29–30.

Dochterman, J. (2006). Effectiveness research: Three examples [Abstracts]. *International Journal of Nursing Terminologies and Classifications, 17* (1), 85–87.

Fehring, R.J. (1986). Validating diagnostic labels: Standardized methodology. In E. Hurley (Ed.), *Classification of nursing diagnoses: Proceedings of the sixth conference* (pp. 183–190). St. Louis, MO: NANDA.

Grant, J.S., Kinney, M., & Guzzetta, C.E. (1990). Using magnitude estimation scaling to examine the validity of nursing diagnoses. *Nursing Diagnosis, 1*(2), 64–69.

Hasegawa, T., Ogaswara, C., Tachibana, S., Hayakawa, M., Ooguchi, F., Ohkita, M., Yonezawa, H., & Tanabe, M. (2006). Validity of written case studies as a tool to measure nurses' ability for making nursing diagnoses. *International Journal of Nursing Terminologies and Classifications, 17,* 36–37.

Kim, M.J., Amoroso-Seritella, R., Gulanick, M., Moyer, K., Parsons, E., Scherbel, J., Staffors, M.J., Suhayda, R., & Yocom, C. (1984). Clinical validation of cardiovascular nursing diagnoses. In M.J. Kim, G.K. McFarland, & A.M. McLane (Eds.), *Classification of nursing diagnoses: Proceedings of the fifth national conference* (pp. 128–138). St. Louis: Mosby.

Lamont, S.C. (2006). Supportive role performance: Development of a new wellness diagnosis [Abstract]. *International Journal of Nursing Terminologies and Classifications, 17* (1), 40–41.

Lunney, M. (2001). *Critical thinking and nursing diagnosis: Case studies and analyses.* Philadelphia: NANDA

Maas, M.L., Hardy, M.A., & Craft, M. (1990). Methodologic considerations in nursing diagnosis research. *Nursing Diagnosis, 1* (1), 24–30.

Minthorn, C.N. (2006). Meeting magnet research criteria with studies of NANDA, NIC and NOC [Abstract]. *International Journal of Nursing Terminologies and Classifications, 17* (1), 46–47.

Parker, L., & Lunney, M. (1998). Moving beyond content validation of nursing diagnosis. *Nursing Diagnosis: The Journal of Nursing Language and Classification, 9,* 144–150.

Sparks, S.M., & Lien-Gieschen, T. (1994). Modification of the diagnostic content validity model. *Nursing Diagnosis, 5* (1), 31–35.

Walker, L.O., & Avant, K.C. (2005). *Strategies for theory construction in nursing* (4th ed.). Upper Saddle River, NJ: Pearson Prentice Hall.

Waltz, C.F., Strickland, O.L., & Lenz, E.R. (2005). *Measurement in nursing and health sciences research* (3rd ed.). New York: Springer.

Welton, J.M., & Halloran, E.J. (2005). Nursing diagnosis, diagnosis-related group, and hospital outcomes. *Journal of Nursing Administration, 35,* 541–549.

Westmoreland, D., Wesorick, B., Hanson, D., & Wyngarden, K. (2000). Consensus validation of clinical practice model practice guidelines. *Journal of Nursing Care Quality, 14*(4), 16–27.

Whitley, G.G. (1992). Concept analysis of fear. *Nursing Diagnosis, 3,* 155–161.

Whitley, G.G. (1999). Processes and methodologies for research validation of nursing diagnoses. *Nursing Diagnosis, 10*(1), 5–14.

Nursing Diagnosis in Administration

Dickon Weir-Hughes, EdD, RN, FRSH

Since the advent of the nursing diagnosis movement in the 1970s, some of the finest nurse scholars have been attracted to support the work. Many of these activists have been clinically focused academics, researchers, and educationals, and some have also been expert clinicians. It is notable, however, that chief nurses/nurse directors, administrators, or managers have generally been less active in this important area of nursing development. This is intriguing because nursing diagnosis is so fundamental to the provision of high quality nursing care and the benefits are so numerous, that it would seem obvious that even the busiest nurse leader would make its development and implementation a priority. In an era when both cost containment and evidence-based practice are key objectives for nurse leaders, classifying, clarifying, and documenting the phenomena that are of professional concern to nurses is essential.

Why Implement Nursing Diagnosis Into a Clinical Environment?

The implementation of nursing diagnosis brings a number of benefits to patient care — improved and more consistent care planning; improved nurse-to-nurse, nurse-to-physician, and nurse-to-patient communication; and better recognition of phenomena that nurses find challenging to assess and describe, such as psychological, spiritual, and sexual issues. From an organizational point of view, nursing diagnosis helps to improve clinical governance and risk management; and clearly demonstrates a commitment to bring together nursing theory, education, and clinical practice — in other words, evidence-based nursing. Importantly, it also enables nurse leaders and researchers to evaluate nursing practice across an organization in a consistent and thought-provoking way.

A number of studies, including those by Halloran and Kiley (1987), published in a range of peer-reviewed journals between 1985 and 1987 examine the whole notion of the use of diagnostic related groups (DRG) and related systems that attach payment to procedures or medical conditions rather than actual patient dependency. Halloran and Kiley examined 1,288 adult medical and surgical patients in an urban teaching hospital in the U.S. The complexity of medical treatment was measured by use of the DRG relative cost weight. The nursing indicator was derived from a set of nursing diagnoses. The study findings found that DRG cost weight is a poor predicator of dependency (and therefore costs of care) and that the nursing-dependency index, based on a series of 61 nursing diagnoses, added significantly to the DRG weight in explaining length of stay and other issues. Given that the nursing resource is one of the most significant areas of expenditure for any healthcare organization and that organizations are frequently reliant on the number of nurses it has available to take in more work, this is a significant finding. The Halloran and Kiley study, and one by Frank and Lave (1985), indicate that to be cost efficient in relation to length of stay, it is essential to include a nursing-dependency factor based on nursing diagnoses in forward planning. It is sobering that 20 years later nurse leaders still have not taken forward the use of nursing diagnosis in ways recommended by these seminal pieces of work.

Evidence-Based Practice: Integrating Theory and Practice

The nursing research and outcomes opportunities that emerge as a result of using nursing diagnosis are phenomenal and unparalleled. Almost 150 years ago Florence Nightingale (1863) commented on the paucity of comparative outcomes data on nursing interventions. "In an attempt to arrive at the truth, I have applied everywhere for information, but in scarcely an instance have I been able to obtain hospital records fit for any purpose of comparison. They would show the subscribers how their money was being spent, what good was really being done with it. They would enable us, besides, to ascertain the influence of the hospital…upon the course of operations and diseases passing through its wards; and the truth thus ascertained would enable us to save life and suffering and to improve the management of the sick" (pp. 175-176).

Although major strides have been made in some places, it is concerning that 150 years later many nursing organizations, whether in hospitals or community settings, are still failing to evaluate their practice in a consistent manner. Nursing diagnosis data collected from clinical areas allow nurses to evaluate their individual clinical practice and explicitly integrate theory and practice. As well, the data allow nurse leaders and researchers to evaluate, audit, and establish practice priorities organizationally through conducting prevalence studies. This information can then help to define the content of inservice education and even university-based educational offerings.

Nursing in the Era of Electronic Patient Records

The essence of nursing is the therapeutic professional relationship between nurse and patient. Although information systems may appear to be cold and literal, there is no reason why an electronic patient records system should do anything but enhance the clinical role of the nurse by saving time and improving documentation. Within some such systems, however, there is a tendency to see nursing reduced to an automated list of tasks generated by standardised care pathways. This reductionist approach to professional nursing is neither clinically safe nor commercially savvy because it ignores the needs of individual patients. Assessing, meeting, and evaluating such individual needs is key to safe patient care and providing the levels of patient satisfaction omnipresent in the ever more consumer-driven health sector in which nurses practice.

It is well-recognised that the implementation of any healthcare information system provides the opportunity to review and improve clinical practice. Unfortunately, it is also recognised that some system implementations have had extremely negative consequences on nursing practice and, therefore, patient care. These consequences are manifested in a variety of ways. From a clinical point of view, poorly planned and under professionally led systems reduce nursing to a care pathway-generated list of tasks that ignores the needs of individuals, and which only serves as a retrograde step to developing patient-focused care. This sort of implementation has been found to give rise to unsafe, unthinking nursing practice, which creates a major clinical governance issue.

From a leadership perspective, systems that radically change nursing practice overnight create enormous problems for clinical staff, who not only have to get used to a new IT system but to numerous new concepts in documenting and planning care, such as using standard nursing language. However, when well-managed and professionally led, there are numerous benefits to bringing together nursing diagnosis and an electronic patient record. Systems that support nursing diagnosis functionality enable nurses to plan care using gold standard, evidence-based nursing. This is key to the reputation of the system vendor and essential for the credibility and legal status of healthcare organisations. From a research and audit perspective, using an electronic patient record based on nursing diagnoses means that comparative data about nursing diagnoses, prevalence, incidence, and linkages to interventions and outcomes can be retrieved quickly and easily. This information can be used to inform an organisation's nursing strategy, workforce design, curriculum planning, and to define in-service education priorities.

Leading the Implementation of Nursing Diagnosis in Clinical Practice

The key nursing diagnosis challenge for nurse leaders is its implementation into everyday clinical practice. Implementation is variable throughout the developed world and even within health systems. However, successful implementation requires expert, high level nursing leadership, ideally at a Board or organisational "top team" level. A range of leadership skills is required for successful implementation—high levels of technical ability, influencing skills, delegation, strategic thinking, networking, and following through. It is vital that nurse leaders thoroughly understand the use and development of nursing diagnosis and can inspire, harness enthusiasm, manage dissent, and answer questions from clinicians with an in-depth understanding of the challenges. As stakeholders in the future of nursing, it is vital to engage nurses at all levels in this important developmental work.

The amount of attention paid to nursing diagnosis in undergraduate nursing programs varies quite significantly worldwide. In terms of inservice education and implementation support, nurses typically need preparation and/or updating in critical thinking and the use of nursing diagnosis and associated assessment tools. Typically, this teaching can be covered in an intensive one- or two- day program with follow-up support in clinical areas from mentors who have this knowledge. Nurses also need paper-based manuals of nursing diagnoses. In many environments, nursing diagnosis is used within electronic patient records and therefore IT training will be required. It is important to understand that teaching nursing diagnosis and critical thinking should be nurse-led, not IT- led, so the focus will be on nursing. Suggested ways of engaging stakeholders and raising awareness include having nursing diagnosis in all regular teaching programs, encouraging attendance at international nursing diagnosis conferences, organising Grand Rounds where cases are presented using nursing diagnosis, and starting focused journal clubs.

Conclusion

Using nursing diagnosis is key to the future of evidence-based, professionally led nursing care. Thus, it needs to be a priority for all nurse leaders in administration and management in order to make nursing practice visible, which is vital to the future of our profession and to enabling us to more effectively meet the needs of patients.

References

Frank, R., & Lave. J. (1985). The psychiatric DRGs: Are they different? *Medical Care, 23,* 1148–1155.

Halloran, E., & Kiley, M. (1987). Nursing dependency, diagnosis-related groups, and length of stay. *Health Care Financing Review, 8*(3), 27–36.

Nightingale , F. (1863). *Notes on hospitals.* London: Longman, Roberts, Green.

NANDA-I Diagnosis Submission Guidelines
Protocol for Submission or Revision of Diagnoses

Proposed diagnoses and revisions of diagnoses undergo a systematic review to determine consistency with the established criteria for a nursing diagnosis. All submissions are subsequently staged according to evidence supporting either the level of development or validation.

Diagnoses may be submitted at various levels of development (e.g., label and definition; label, definition, defining characteristics or risk factors, and related factors). All submissions must include supporting references. Indicate if no nursing literature is available. Related research from other disciplines is also appropriate to include.

Articles used for the submssion are to be catalogued in the reference section of the submission form.

NANDA-I Diagnosis Submission Guidelines are available on the NANDA-I Web site (www.nanda.org) and the NLINKS Web site (www.nlinks.org; click on "diagnostic review"). Diagnoses may be submitted electronically using the form available on the NANDA-I Web site. Submissions not submitted electroncially should be sent as an e-mail attachment to info@nanda.org, using the format provided on the NANDA-I Web site.

On receipt, the diagnosis will be assigned to a primary reviewer from the Diagnosis Development Committee (DDC). This person will work with the submitter as the DDC reviews the submission. At this point, the submission will also be identified on the NANDA-I Web site as a submission in review.

Full Review Process

New diagnoses go through *a full review process,* which includes the following steps:

1. Posting on the NANDA-I Web site

2. Review of submission by the primary reviewer

3. Primary reviewer works with submitter to address changes that need to be made

4. Submission is forwarded to full DDC for review.

5. DDC recommends one of the following:
   a. Approve with no recommendations
   b. Approve pending follow-through with recommendations (most frequent DDC decision)
   c. Disapprove

6. The primary reviewer forwards the DDC recommendations to the submitter and works with the submitter to make the recommended changes.

7. Submissions approved by the DDC are presented and discussed at the biennial conference in order to invite extended member input. Recommendations from the forums are reviewed with the submitter and by the DDC.

8. The submission is then forwarded to the NANDA International Board of Directors for final approval. Diagnoses accepted at the 2.1 level of development will be incorporated into both the NANDA-I Taxonomy and the NNN Taxonomy of Nursing Practice, and published in the next edition of *NANDA-I Nursing Diagnoses: Definitions & Classification.*

New Diagnosis Submission Process

To submit a new diagnosis for consideration by the DDC, follow these steps:

1. Obtain the most recent edition of *NANDA-I Nursing Diagnoses: Definitions and Classification* and review related diagnoses in the book. Refer to the NANDA-I Diagnosis Sub-

mission Guidelines on the NANDA-I Web site (www. nanda.org) and the NLINKS Web site (www.nlinks.org; click on "diagnostic review"). Follow the guidelines on the Web in case they have been updated since publication of the most recent edition of the NANDA-I book.

2. Contact Leann Scroggins (scroggins.leann@mayo.edu), Chair of the DDC, for more specific instructions, guidelines regarding format, criteria for assigning level of evidence, and protocol for submission.

3. Review "Glossary of Terms" in the most recent edition of *NANDA-I Nursing Diagnoses: Definitions and Classification.*

4. Decide whether your diagnosis is an actual diagnosis, risk diagnosis, wellness diagnosis, or health-promotion diagnosis.

5. Provide a label for the diagnosis.

6. Provide a definition for the diagnosis that is supported by references. Identify the references.

7. Identify the defining characteristics or risk factors for the diagnosis. Actual diagnoses, wellness diagnoses, and health-promotion diagnoses have defining characteristics; risk diagnoses have risk factors. To facilitate coding, each defining characteristic and risk factor must contain a single concept rather than multiple concepts. For example, rather than listing "nausea & vomiting" as a single defining characteristic or risk factor, each one needs to be listed separately. References (articles, not books) to back up each defining characteristic or risk factor are required and must be identified. The references should be research-based, if possible. If no research-based references or nursing references are available, indicate this in your submission.

8. Identify related factors for actual diagnoses. To facilitate coding, related factors must be single concepts, not multiple concepts. Risk diagnoses, wellness diagnoses, and health-promotion diagnoses do not have related factors. References are required for each related factor and must be identified.

9. Develop a bibliography, including all the articles referenced. Number the references and link the reference to the component(s) of your submission the reference supports. In addition, **boldface** or place an asterisk by the three key references you want to be included in the next edition of *NANDA-I Nursing Diagnoses: Definitions and Classification* when your submission is accepted.

10. Provide examples of appropriate nursing interventions (may be NIC or other nursing interventions) and nursing outcomes (may be NOC or other nursing outcomes) for the diagnosis.

11. Use the electronic submission process available on the NANDA-I Web site or e-mail your submission to info@nanda.org.

12. You will be notified when your work has been received and will be given an estimate of the time it will take before you can expect to receive a response from the DDC. Most submissions need some additional work for refinement. You will be assigned a mentor from the DDC to assist you through the process.

Diagnosis Revision Process

To submit a revision of a current diagnosis for consideration by the DDC, follow these steps:

1. Obtain the most recent edition of *NANDA-I Nursing Diagnoses: Definitions and Classification* and review related diag-

noses in the book. Refer to the NANDA-I Diagnosis Submission Guidelines on the NANDA-I Web site (www.nanda.org) and the NLINKS Web site (www.nlinks.org; click on "diagnostic review"). Follow the guidelines on the Web in case they have been updated since publication of the most recent edition of the NANDA-I book.

2. Contact Leann Scroggins (scroggins.leann@mayo.edu), Chair DDC, for more specific instructions, guidelines regarding format, criteria for assigning level of evidence, and protocol for submission.

3. Review "Glossary of Terms" in the most recent edition of *NANDA-I Nursing Diagnoses: Definitions and Classification.*

4. Identify if the label of the diagnosis needs revision.

5. Review the definition of the diagnosis to determine if revision is necessary; revise if appropriate. The revision must be supported by references and the references must be identified.

6. Review the defining characteristics or risk factors for the diagnosis. Actual diagnoses, wellness diagnoses, and health-promotion diagnoses have defining characteristics; risk diagnoses have risk factors. To facilitate coding, each defining characteristic and risk factor must contain a single concept rather than multiple concepts. For example, rather than listing "nausea & vomiting" as a single defining characteristic or risk factor, list each one separately. Identify the appropriate changes in the defining characteristics or risk factors and support each change with references. References (articles, not books) to back up each defining characteristic or risk factor are required and must be identified. The references should be research-based, if possible. If no research-based references or nursing references are available, indicate this in your submission.

7. Review the related factors for the actual diagnosis. To facilitate coding, related factors must be single concepts, not multiple concepts. Risk diagnoses, wellness diagnoses, and health-promotion diagnoses do not have related factors. References are required for each related factor and must be identified.

8. Develop a bibliography, including all articles referenced. Number the references and link the reference to the component(s) of your submission the reference supports. In addition, **boldface** or place an asterisk by the three key references you want to be included in *NANDA-I Nursing Diagnoses: Definitions and Classification* when your submission is accepted.

9. If the revision is changing the original intent of the diagnosis, provide examples of appropriate nursing interventions (may be NIC or other nursing interventions) and nursing outcomes (may be NOC or other nursing outcomes) for the diagnosis.

10. Use the electronic submission process available on the NANDA International Web or e-mail your submission to info@nanda.org.

11. You will be notified when your work has been received and given an estimate of the time it will take before you can expect to receive a response from the DDC. Revised diagnoses may undergo a full review process or an expedited review process, depending on the extent of revisions being proposed. The DDC will make this decision and tell you which process is needed. Most submissions need some additional work for refinement. You will be assigned a mentor from the DDC to assist you through the process.

Expedited Review Process

An expedited review process (ERP) is appropriate only for proposed revisions of current diagnoses. The ERP is a streamlined process intended to facilitate rapid review of proposed revisions of diagnoses when the proposed revisions are considered by the DDC to be minor in nature and do not alter the original intent of the diagnoses. Examples of such revisions may include:

- Editing and clarification of definition
- Limited addition of defining characteristics or related factors

An ERP includes the following steps:

1. Posting on the NANDA-I Web site

2. Review of submission by the primary reviewer

3. Primary reviewer works with submitter to address needed changes that need to be made

4. Submission is forwarded to the DDC for review.

5. DDC recommends one of the following:
   a. Approve with no recommendations
   b. Approve pending follow-through with recommendations (most frequent DDC decision)
   c. Disapprove

6. The primary reviewer forwards the DDC recommendations to the submitter and works with the submitter to make the recommended changes.

7. Submissions approved by the DDC are forwarded to the NANDA-I Board of Directors for approval. Approval of the proposed revision is posted on the NANDA-I Web site.

NANDA-I Diagnosis Submission: Level of Evidence Criteria

1 Received for Development (Consultation from DDC)

1.1 Label Only

This level is intended primarily for submission by organized groups rather than individuals. The DDC will consult with the submitter and provide education related to diagnostic development through printed guidelines and workshops. At this stage the label is categorized as "received for development" and identified as such on the NANDA-I Web site and in *NANDA-I Nursing Diagnoses: Definitions and Classification.*

1.2 Label and Definition

The label is clear and stated at a basic level. The definition is consistent with the label. The label and definition are distinct from other NANDA-I diagnoses and definitions. The definition differs from the defining characteristics and label, and these components are not included in the definition. At this stage, the diagnosis must be consistent with the current NANDA-I definition of nursing diagnosis (page 332). The definition is supported by literature references and these are identified.

1.3 Label, Definition, and Defining Characteristics or Risk Factors

The defining characteristics or risk factors (for risk diagnoses) are consistent with the label. The defining characteristics or risk factors are distinct, observable, and measurable. Each defining characteristic and risk factor contains a single concept rather than a listing of multiple concepts, and each one is supported by literature references and these are identified. The content is consistent with all NANDA-I definitions and qualifiers.

2 Accepted for Publication and Inclusion in the NANDA-I Taxonomy and the NNN Nursing Practice Taxonomy

2.1 Label, Definition, Defining Characteristics or Risk Factors, Related Factors, and References

At 2.1, references are cited for the definition, each defining characteristic or risk factor, and each related factor. In addition, it is recommended that the submitter provide examples of nursing interventions (NIC or other nursing intervention) and nursing outcomes (NOC or other nursing outcome). The label will be forwarded to the Taxonomy Committee for classification.

2.2 Concept Analysis

The criteria in 2.1 are met. In addition, a narrative review of relevant literature, culminating in a written concept analysis, is required to demonstrate the existence of a substantive body of knowledge underlying the diagnosis. The literature review/concept analysis supports the label and definition, and includes discussion and support of the defining characteristics or risk factors (for risk diagnoses) and related factors (for actual diagnoses).

2.3 Consensus Studies Related to Diagnosis Using Experts

The criteria in 2.2 are met. Studies include those soliciting expert opinion, Delphi, and similar studies of diagnostic components in which nurses are subjects.

3 Clinically Supported (Validation and Testing)

3.1 Literature Synthesis

The criteria in 2.2 are met. The synthesis is in the form of an integrated review of the literature. Search terms/MESH terms used in the review are provided to assist future researchers.

3.2 Clinical Studies Related to Diagnosis, But Not Generalizable to the Population

The criteria in 2.2 are met. The narrative includes a description of studies related to the diagnosis, which includes defining characteristics or risk factors, and related factors. Studies may be qualitative in nature, or quantitative studies using nonrandom samples in which patients are subjects.

3.3 Well-Designed Clinical Studies With Small Sample Sizes

The criteria in 2.2 are met. The narrative includes a description of studies related to the diagnosis, which includes defining characteristics or risk factors. Random sampling is used in these studies, but the sample size is limited.

3.4 Well-Designed Clinical Studies With Random Sample of Sufficient Size to Allow for Generalizability to the Overall Population

The criteria in 2.2 are met. The narrative includes a description of studies related to the diagnosis, which includes defining characteristics or risk factors, and related factors. Random sampling is used in these studies and the sample size is sufficient to allow for generalizability of results to the overall population.

Procedure to Appeal a DDC Decision on Diagnosis Review

If a diagnosis/revision is reviewed by the DDC and returned to the submitter(s) either for revision or because it is judged not to meet one or more criteria for staging a diagnosis, the submitter(s) may appeal the decision.

If the DDC chooses not to accept a diagnosis/revision, notification of nonacceptance will be given to the submitter(s) with detailed rationale. One or more of the following reasons will be explained:

■ Reject diagnosis (e.g., does not meet criteria for the definition of a nursing diagnosis or does not meet diagnosis level of evidence criteria)

■ Return with substantial revision (e.g., need to make major content changes)

■ Insufficient/old literature support (e.g., failure to reference meta analyses, concept papers, current research, or lack of research articles)

■ Return with editorial changes (e.g., solicit submitter response to DDC rationale and/or revision to submission)

If the submitter(s) choose(s) to appeal the DDC decision, the proposed diagnosis/revision will be placed on the NANDA International Web site (www.nanda.org) and will be announced in the journal. A period of 90 days will be provided for members to submit evidence supporting, modifying, or rejecting the diagnosis/revision. After 90 days, the DDC will review feedback and submit a second decision to the submitter(s).

If the DDC chooses not to accept a diagnosis following the second review, the submitter(s) will have an opportunity at the biennial conference to present the diagnosis/revision and the rationale for disagreement with the DDC decision. The presentation will occur in an open session and require evidence-based argument from the submitter(s) and the DDC regarding the decision. Conference attendees will also have the opportunity to present evidence-based argument supporting, modifying, or rejecting the diagnosis/revision.

Following the open session, the DDC will review all information and forward a decision to the submitter(s) and the Board of Directors.

The NANDA International Board of Directors will have an opportunity to provide evidence-based argument supporting, modifying, or rejecting the submission at two points:

1. During the open forum at the biennial conference.
2. After the conference, the Board of Directors will provide a final review of the DDC recommendation for approval. A decision by the Board of Directors to modify or reject the DDC's recommendation must be evidence-based and at the same LOE or higher as the evidence presented by the submitter(s) and/or by the DDC.

Glossary of Terms

Nursing Diagnoses

Nursing diagnosis A clinical judgment about individual, family, or community responses to actual or potential health problems/life processes. A nursing diagnosis provides the basis for selection of nursing interventions to achieve outcomes for which the nurse is accountable (approved at the 9th conference, 1990).

Actual nursing diagnosis Describes human responses to health conditions/life processes that exist in an individual, family, or community. It is supported by defining characteristics (manifestations, signs and symptoms) that cluster in patterns of related cues or inferences.

Health-promotion nursing diagnosis Clinical judgment of a person's, family's, or community's motivation and desire to increase well-being and actualize human health potential as expressed in their readiness to enhance specific health behaviors such as nutrition and exercise. Health-promotion diagnoses can be used in any health state and do not require current levels of wellness. This readiness is supported by defining characteristics. Interventions are selected in concert with the individual/family/community to best ensure the ability to reach the stated outcomes.

Risk nursing diagnosis Describes human responses to health conditions/life processes that may develop in a vulnerable individual, family, or community. It is supported by risk factors that contribute to increased vulnerability.

Syndrome "A cluster or group of signs and symptoms that almost always occur together. Together, these clusters represent a distinct clinical picture" (McCourt, 1991, p. 79).

Wellness nursing diagnosis Describes human responses to levels of wellness in an individual, family, or community that have a readiness for enhancement. This readiness is supported by defining characteristics. As with all diagnoses, nurse-sensitive (sensitive to nursing interventions) outcomes are identified and nursing interventions are selected that will provide a high likelihood of reaching the outcomes.

Components of a Diagnosis

Label Provides a name for a diagnosis. It is a concise term or phrase that represents a pattern of related cues. It may include modifiers.

Definition Provides a clear, precise description; delineates its meaning and helps differentiate it from similar diagnoses.

Defining characteristics Observable cues/inferences that cluster as manifestations of an actual or wellness nursing diagnosis.

Risk factors Environmental factors and physiological, psychological, genetic, or chemical elements that increase the vulnerability of an individual, family, or community to an unhealthful event.

Related factors Factors that appear to show some type of patterned relationship with the nursing diagnosis. Such factors may be described as antecedent to, associated with, related to, contributing to, or abetting. Only actual nursing diagnoses have related factors.

Definitions for Classification of Nursing Diagnoses

Classification Systematic arrangement of related phenomena in groups or classes based on characteristics that objects have in common

Level of abstraction Describes the concreteness/abstractness of a concept:

(a) Very abstract concepts are theoretical, may not be directly measurable, defined by concrete concepts, inclusive of concrete concepts, disassociated from any specific instance, independent of time and space, have more general descriptors, may not be clinically useful for planning treatment.

(b) Concrete concepts are observable and measurable, limited by time and space, constitute a specific category, more exclusive, name a real thing or class of things, restricted by nature, may be clinically useful for planning treatment.

Nomenclature A system of designations (terms) elaborated according to pre-established rules (American Nurses Association, 1999)

Taxonomy Classification according to presumed natural relationships among types and their subtypes (American Nurses Association, 1999).

References

American Nurses Association. (1999). *ANA CNP II recognition criteria and definitions.* Washington, DC: Author.

McCourt, A. (1991). In R.M. Carroll-Johnson (Ed.), *Classification of nursing diagnoses: Proceedings of the ninth conference* (p. 79). Philadelphia: Lippincott.

2007–2008

NANDA International Board of Directors

President: T. Heather Herdman, PhD, RN
President-Elect: Dickon Weir-Hughes, EdD, RN, FRSH
Treasurer: Anne Perry, EdD, RN, FAAN
Directors:
Jane Brokel, PhD, RN
Dame June Clark, PhD, RN, RHV, FRNC, DBE
Leann Scroggins, MS, RN, CRRN-A, APRN BC
Gunn Von Krogh, RN

NANDA International Diagnosis Development Committee

Leann Scroggins, MS, RN, CRRN-A, APRN BC, Chair
Lynda Juall Carpenito-Moyet, MSN, RN, CPNP
Crystal Heath, MSN, RN
Dorothy Jones, EdD, RN, FAAN
Shigemi Kamatsura, PhD, RN
Marlene Lindeman, MSN, RN, CS
Sara Lister, MSc, RN, PGDAE
Margaret Lunney, PhD, RN, FAAN
Meridean Maas, PhD, RN, FAAN
Geralyn Meyer, PhD, RN
Lina Rahal, MEd, RN

NANDA International Taxonomy Committee

Barbara Vassallo, EdD, RN, CS, ANPC, Chair
Sally Decker, PhD, RN
Carme Espinosa, RN
J. Adolf Guirao Goris, RN
Marion Johnson, PhD, RN
Mikyoung Lee, PhD, RN
Carol Soares O'Hearn, PhD, RN, CPRQ
Elizabeth Rose, PhD, RN

An Invitation to Join NANDA International

Mission

To advance the development of nursing terminologies and classifications and provide nurses at all levels of practice with a standardized language to:

- Assess client responses to actual or potential health problems or life crises,
- Document care for reimbursement of nursing services by third party insurers, and
- Create and use databases that facilitate documentation and study of the phenomena of concern to nurses in order to improve patient care.

Functions

1. Provide nurses with a standardized language describing their practice that can be used to communicate with nurses across all specialties and cultures, members of other healthcare disciplines, and the healthcare consumer.
2. Provide a system for developing, validating, and refining nursing terminologies and classifications.
3. Publish a quarterly journal that contains the latest thinking about nursing terminologies and classifications worldwide.
4. Provide support, communication, and resources through conferences, publications, funding, and networking. Mentoring is available for nurses who are interested in developing new diagnoses and refining current diagnoses.

Membership Requirements

Membership is open to all registered nurses with a current RN license. Associate membership is extended to nonregistered nurses and students who share an interest in the purpose of the association. Institutional membership is extended to those associations and organizations that believe in and want to support the mission of NANDA International.

Organizational Background

The North American Nursing Diagnosis Association (NANDA) was founded in 1982, replacing the National Conference Group that was established in 1973. In 2002 the association name was changed to NANDA International to reflect its worldwide expansion. To date, NANDA-I has approved 188 diagnoses for clinical testing and refinement.

A dynamic process of diagnosis review and taxonomy development continues toward identifying and classifying nursing phenomena. NANDA-I approved diagnoses are included in the Unified Medical Language System of the National Library of Medicine and Health Level 7 (HL7), and NANDA-I is working with the American Nurses Association to develop a Unified Nursing Language System. NANDA-I is also cooperating with the International Council of Nurses to develop an International Classification of Nursing Practice.

Benefits of Membership

1. Subscription to the *International Journal of Nursing Terminologies and Classifications*
2. Reduced registration fee at the biennial conference.
3. Participation in decisions about new and revised diagnoses.
4. State-of-the-art information on development of nursing language systems, which enable nurses to communicate with one another around the world.
5. Reduced rate on in-house publications, such as *NANDA-I Nursing Diagnoses: Definitions & Classification.*
6. Resources for networking and research data.
7. Access to the NANDA-I Web page with links to minutes from the Board of Director meetings and all current decisions and initiatives.

Joint membership is available for members of ACENDIO and AENTDE at time of publishing. Contact the NANDA-I office to see if a joint membership is available with other organizations related to standardized nursing language to which you belong.

Additional Materials Available

NANDA-I publishes its taxonomy in *NANDA-I Nursing Diagnoses: Definitions and Classification.* A new edition is printed after each biennial conference. This book contains the only list of diagnoses approved by NANDA-I for distribution.

To order or obtain information on NANDA-I publications or conferences, contact the NANDA-I office:
100 N. 20th Street, 4th Floor, Philadelphia, PA, 19103, USA.
800.647.9002; E-mail: info@nanda.org;
Web: www.nanda.org

Membership Committee

Kay Avant, PhD, RN, FAAN, Chair
Carme Espinosa
Sharie Falan, PhD, RN
Teresa A. Garcia, MSN, RN
Sara Lister, MSc, RN, PGDAE
Jayne Hansche Lobert, MS, APRN, NP, BC
Regena Soyer
Alexandra M. Westbrook

☐YES! I WANT TO SUPPORT THE NURSING TERMINOLOGY MOVEMENT. PLEASE ACCEPT MY APPLICATION FOR NANDA INTERNATIONAL MEMBERSHIP:

☐Regular Membership (RNs only)...US $105*
☐Retired Membership ....US $ 65*
☐Associate Membership (non-RNs welcome) ....US $105*
☐Student Membership ....US $ 35*

Institutional membership is also available. For details contact: info@nanda.org

☐Send ___copy(ies) of *NANDA-I Nursing Diagnoses*: $_____
   Definitions & Classification at special member's price:
   US $19.95/ea. (non-members, $24.95)

☐Send ___copy(ies) of *Critical Thinking & Nursing* $_____
   Diagnoses at special member's price: US $19.95/ea.

☐I am also enclosing my tax-deductible donation to $_____
   the NANDA-I Foundation

TOTAL ENCLOSED ....U.S. $_____

NANDA's Federal Tax ID # is 41-1363777.

☐Check enclosed   ☐Money order enclosed
   (Payable to NANDA-I. U.S. funds drawn on U.S. banks only)
☐Charge my credit card: ☐AmEx   ☐MC   ☐Visa
   CARD # _____
   Signature_____ Exp. date___/___

* U.S. $29 of this amount is for your one-year subscription to the *International Journal of Nursing Terminologies & Classifications*.

PLEASE PRINT

_____
FIRST NAME   M.I.

_____
LAST NAME & CREDENTIALS

_____
CURRENT LICENSE NUMBER

_____
POSITION/TITLE(S)

_____
COMPANY/INSTITUTION

_____
DEPARTMENT

_____
MAILING ADDRESS (PREFERRED) _ HOME _ BUSINESS

_____
CITY

_____
STATE/PROVINCE   ZIP/POSTAL CODE   COUNTRY

_____
TELEPHONE   FAX

_____
E-MAIL ADDRESS

Who referred you to NANDA International?_____
U.S.-Registered RNs only: Are you an ANA Member?   ☐Yes   ☐No
What is your clinical specialty?

_____

☐Please remove my name from rented mail lists.

Index

Notes